Health in Saudi Arabia

Vol. One

Health in Saudi Arabia

Vol. One

2nd Edition

Zohair A. Sebai

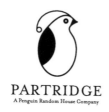

PARTRIDGE
A Penguin Random House Company

To order additional copies of this book, contact
Toll Free 800 101 2657 (Singapore)
Toll Free 1 800 81 7340 (Malaysia)
orders.singapore@partridgepublishing.com

www.partridgepublishing.com/singapore

Contents

Preface

There has been always a pressing need for a book which presents health topics in Saudi Arabia to planners, educators, learners and medical practitioners. This book tries to fulfill part of this need.

Volume I, an introduction and perspective, discusses some features of health problems, health manpower and medical education in Saudi Arabia. It also provides under and post-graduate medical students with material for problem based learning.

Volume II, which is under writing, discusses aspects of health resources, problems and services in the country.

The book in its two volumes is far from being complete or comprehensive. It gives base line information on health in a country which is developing very fast and still virgin in medical research.

Acknowledgment

The material in this book is based mostly on fieldworks carried out in various parts of the Kingdom. To all my colleagues, students and assistants who participated in the fieldwork I extend a special word of gratitude.

I wish to thank Professor David Price Evans and Professor Herbert M. Gilles for their constructive comments. The great assistance given by Messrs. Brian Duffy and Eddie R. Musngi in typing the manuscript on the word processor and Mr. Chris Smith and Miss Hoda Sharabash in reviewing and editing made the writing a pleasant task.

بسم الله الرحمن الرحيم

مقدمـــــــة

بين يدي القارىء الكريم الجزء الأول من كتاب الصحة في المملكة العربية السعودية وسوف يليه الجزء الثاني إن شاء الله. الكتاب يحاول أن يسد بعض الفراغ الذي نجده في المعلومات الصحية في بلادنا. وهو موجه أساسا للأطباء وطلبة الطب وطلبة الدراسات الطبية العليا وإلى جميع المهتمين بالتعليم الطبي والخدمات الصحية.

الجزء الأول يستعرض بضع قضايا أساسية تعد مدخلاً لنقاش الوضع الصحي في المملكة كما أنه يلقي بعض الضوء على عدة بدائل للارتفاع بالوضع الصحي فيها.

في الفصول الأولى من هذا الجزء استعرضنا بعض المشاكل الصحية في دول العالم النامي ـ والمملكة واحدة منها وان كانت سريعة الخطى في نموها ـ وخلصنا من هذه الفصول الى أن لدى كثير من دول العالم النامي امكانيات مادية وبشرية كافية تستطيع إن أحسن استغلالها أن تنهض بالمستوى الصحي أفضل نهوض. ومن الواجب على هذه الدول أن تستفيد من التقنية الحديثة التي ابتدعتها الدول المتقدمة صناعيا في مجالات التعليم الصحي والرعاية الصحية على شرط أن توجهها بما يتلاءم مع احتياجاتها وامكاناتها ولا تنقلها من مصادرها بشكل عشوائي. ويكفينا مثلا على ذلك التعليم الطبي فقد ورثت كثير من الدول النامية مناهجه من الغرب ومن ثم ركزت اهتمامها على تعليم الأطباء داخل المستشفيات وفي صالات المحاضرات وأهملت أشد الاهمال اتصال الدارسين بالمشاكل الصحية في البيئة وتدر بهم على الوقاية من أسباب الأمراض.

وفى الفصول التالية من الكتاب عرضنا لجوانب من المشاكل الصحية في المملكة من خلال الدراسات الحقلية التي أجريت في بعض المجتمعات الريفية والبدوية مثل تربة البقوم وقرى عسير وخليص والقصيم وغامد وزهران وجيزان. هذه الدراسات الحقلية تلقي الضوء على أسباب المشاكل الصحية في بلادنا كما أنها تعطي بدائل للارتفاع بالمستوى الصحي في هذه المجتمعات خاصة وفي المملكة عامة.

أما الفصول الأخيرة فانها تستعرض قضايا التعليم الطبي والرعاية الصحية الأولية ودور المستشفيات في تطوير الصحة وواقع ومستقبل القوى البشرية في القطاع الصحي. والنتيجة التي تنتهي اليها هذه الفصول هي أن مستقبل الرعاية الصحية في بلادنا يعتمد في الدرجة الأولى على اعداد الفريق الطبي المتكامل واعطاء الجوانب الوقائية حقها من الاهتمام جنبا الى جنب مع العلاج وتطوير الرعاية الصحية الأولية.

وقد كتب الفصلان الأخيران باللغة العربية الأول يدعو الى البدء في تعليم الطب في العالم العربي باللغة
ربية والثاني يدعو الى أن لانتبع في مناهجنا التعليمية في كليات الطب بالعالم العربي مناهج التعليم في
نرب. وقد يتساءل البعض .. كيف تدعو الى تعليم الطب باللغة العربية وتقدم كتابك هذا باللغة الانجليزية
جيب بأن هناك ضرورة أراها ملحة لسد بعض الفراغ الذي نعانيه ووسيلتنا في ذلك ـ مرحليا ـ اللغة
نجليزية. وأرجو أن أفرغ إن شاء الله لترجمته الى اللغة العربية أو قد يتصدى لذلك مشكوراً أحد الأخوة
ملاء.

وفي النهاية أحب أن أشير الى أن بعض فصول هذا الكتاب سبق أن نشرت متفرقة في بعض الكتب أو
بلات العلمية وأعيدت صياغتها هنا. كما أن كثيراً من الزملاء الكرام شاركوا في هذه الدراسات الحقلية
هم واجب الشكر والامتنان. و يسعدني أن أحيي المسئولين في بلادي على على تطلعاتهم الدائمة نحو رعاية صحية
ضل وعلى مايبذلونه من جهد متواصل في هذا السبيل. وأسأل الله أن يوفقنا جميعا لما يحبه و يرضاه.

Introduction

During the last decade Saudi Arabia has experienced a rapid development which is probably unsurpassed by any other nation. It has been a historical phenomenon. The government revenues from oil and other sources recorded an almost 40-fold increase, rising from SR 5.7 billion in 1970 to SR 211 billion in 1980 (US$1 equals SR 3.5). In the same period of time the total number of schools increased from 3,100 to more than 11,000, representing an average annual growth of 14.5 percent. The number of hospital beds increased from 9,039 to 17,523 and the number of physicians increased from 1,172 to 6,461. (The natural population growth is estimated at 2.8 percent per year).

The expansion of health services has brought medical care to almost every village in the country. The rapid growth in economy, health care facilities, urbanization and mass media have changed, in one way or another, health knowledge, attitude and practices of the people.

In spite of the dramatic development in the health sector, some problems remain. The physical development has not been complimented in this short period of time by a parallel development in the national human resources. The expatriate health personnel face cultural and language barriers, especially in rural areas. Information on the magnitude and distribution of health problems and resources are sporadic and incomplete.

Health services remain predominantly curative. Most of the health personnel are products of patient-oriented, hospital-based medical institutes, and the people's demand, as expected, is for curative care.

This book in its two volumes has been written because of the scarcity of health information in Saudi Arabia. It also provides educational material on problem-based learning. The book is written for physicians, medical students and health personnel in general.

Volume One is an Introduction to Health in Saudi Arabia. It also provides postgraduate and undergraduate medical students with material for problem-based learning. This approach promotes self-learning and positive participation on the part of the students. Some of the topics in this volume have already been published as articles in Medical journals and books and have been modified to suit the purpose. Volume Two, "Health in Saudi Arabia; Problems, Services and Resources," discussed the past, present and future of health in Saudi Arabia and is expected to be published in 1986.

Saudi Arabia, as a developing country, needs to exchange experiences with other countries. However, the solution to its problems should be relevant to its own needs and resources, a concept which must always direct medica education and health services systems.

We hope these two volumes will provide the reader with basic knowledge or health in Saudi Arabia and will be a stimulant for discussions and critical views.

ZOHAIR SEBAI

Terms of Reference

Some terms, such as "development," "health," "health standards," "international health," and "epidemiology" are frequently referred to in the text and require common understanding of their meanings.

DEVELOPMENT

Someone, somewhere, invented the terms "developed" and "developing" countries. The issue is controversial. Any country should constantly be "developing," otherwise it becomes stagnant. There are some countries, however, which are more developed economically than others. Nevertheless, an economically developed country might be less developed when it comes to family ties and social justice. In this book, and for the sake of argument, development will be considered in reference to economic status.

HEALTH

Health has been defined by the World Health Organization as "the state of complete physical, mental and social-being and not merely the absence of disease or infirmity."

Hanlon[1] has considered the multifaceted relationships of health and public health in the following terms: "Health is a state of total effective physiological and psychological functioning; it has both a relative and absolute meaning, varying through time and space, both in the individual and in the group; it is the result of the combination of many factors, intrinsic and extrinsic, inherited and contrived, individual and collective, private and public, medical, environmental and social; and it is conditioned by culture, economy, law and government."

PUBLIC HEALTH

The term public health, preventive medicine and hygiene are being used synonymously. Webster's New World Dictionary defines hygiene as "the science of health and its maintenance; system of principles for the preservation of health and prevention of diseases." Preventive medicine is defined as "anything that prevents disease; those people considered together because of some common interest or purpose."

The early concept of public health was limited to sanitary measures Gradually it came to be regarded as an integration of sanitary science and medical science. It has more recently come to be regarded as a sociomedical science.[2]

Winslow[3] in 1920 defined public health as "the science and art of preventing disease, prolonging life and promoting health and efficiency through organized community efforts." He listed the public health activities as "sanitation, control of communicable infections, education, early diagnosis, medical services and the development of social machinery all together to enable every citizen to realize his birthright of health and longevity." The Alma Ata Act in 1978[4] was a repurcussion of the Winslow statement in 1920.

Gershenson[5] summarized the scope of function of public health as follows, "Public health provides a framework to deal with social illness, to alter the ecology, and to make constructive use of all the necessary disciplines. The hierarchial medical model had its time and place: it is dysfunctional in dealing with social illness."

Curative medicine concerns itself with damages already done to an individual, whereas preventive medicine concerns itself with prevention of such damages and promotion of health. There is no line of demarcation between curative and preventive medicine. They are rather a continuity and should always be taken as an integral entity.

In the 1960s the term "community health" was adopted by many medical schools in place of "public health." The term emphasizes the contribution of medical science to public health and implies that the community is the focus of interest.

In the 1970s family medicine emerged as a new specialty which regards the family as an integral unit. More recently the term family and community medicine became popular. It bridges the gap between clinical medicine and public health.

HEALTH INDICES

There are no golden rules on how health standards of a population should be measured. A common practice is, however, to measure health in a community by using certain indices such as the ratio of hospital beds and health personnel to population. These are simple convenient indices, but carry their own biases since they do not reflect the degree of utilization of distribution. In addition they represent means rather than ends. Better indicators of the health standard are the rates of morbidity and mortality.

Infant mortality rate (IMR), Is a sensitive index of the health situation and standard of living in a community. It reflects the impact of hereditary, socioeconomic situation, life style and environmental factors on health.

Neonatal deaths (0-28 days) reflect heredity, ethnicity, maternity condition and prenatal trauma, whereas post neonatal deaths (1-12 months) reflect mostly the effect of environmental factors. The ratio of neonatal deaths to post-neonatal deaths is a sensitive index to the standard of living in the community; the higher the ratio the better the standard.

Perinatal mortality rate (from the 28th week of pregnancy to the first week of life) is another sensitive measure of health. It reflects maternity condition, congenital defects and antenatal and neonatal care. In developed countries the number of deaths during this period exceeds the number of deaths during the first 30 years of life.

The problem in most developing countries is that data on morbidity and mortality may not be accurate or complete.

INTERNATIONAL HEALTH

In modern days the world appears as if it were one community without boundaries, thanks to advanced technology and cultural invasion. The human species is, at least, facing one possible destiny. Every individual's share of the nuclear weapons stockpile equals 3.6 tons of dynamite!

The world community, however, remains divided into subgroups by ethnicity, languages, religious belief, cultural patterns and often prejudices. People still need to learn how to adapt and justly share the heritage of humanity. They, in every sense, have one ancestry, live in one universe and face a common destiny. International health plays a role in strengthening human bonds in health issues.

Tayler[6] defines international health as "the science which includes all types of care in which governments, institutions or individuals from two or more countries share activities or information. It is not a discipline in itself but draws on a wide range of disciplines including all public health specialties, economics, social sciences, planning and management and a broad understanding of ecology."

Malaria, for instance, cannot be controlled in Saudi Arabia unless complementary action takes place in the Gulf region and the Yemen. The same applies to other border-crossing diseases such as cholera, plague, schistosomiasis and tuberculosis. The smallpox eradication program is a good example of how common goals can be achieved by international cooperation. The global eradication program costed less than one year's expenditure on smallpox vaccination in developed countries.

EPIDEMIOLOGY

Epidemiology is the tool of public health planning, implementation and evaluation. The word epidemiology is derived from Greek roots ("epi" means upon, "demos" means people and "logos" means science). The science concerns itself with the study of patterns of diseases and physiological phenomena in human population and the factors influencing these patterns. It discusses these patterns in relation to age, sex, race, occupation, socioeconomic status, place of residence, susceptibility, exposure to specific agents or whatever other characteristic is pertinent.

Descriptive epidemiology tries to answer the questions "who, what, where and when?" (hypothesis generation). Analytic epidemiology builds upon the description and interprets the findings in the light of biologic, genetic and physiologic characteristics, answering the question, why? (hypothesis testing).

Epidemiological studies played a significant role in the evolution of medical sciences and the control of major health problems. The Hippocratic work on airs, waters and places, stressed the importance of environment as a factor in diseases. Al Razi was the first to differentiate between measles and smallpox and the progression of epidemiological knowledge over centuries led to the global eradication of smallpox and the control of measles in many countries.

John Snow's analysis of cholera mortality in London in 1849 (antedating knowledge of bacteriology) led to his implication that polluted water was the vehicle of the "morbid poison." Epidemiological studies by Villerme in the 1820's and Chadwick in the 1840's showed the relationship of poverty to mortality and contributed to the social reform movements in Europe.

The establishment of the germ theory of disease, together with laboratory sciences, provided a base of expansion of epidemiology and the conquest of major epidemic diseases[7].

BIBLIOGRAPHY

1. Hanlon JJ, Picket GE. Pulic Health Administration and Practice. 8th ed. St. Louis: Times Mirror/Mosby, 1984:5.

2. Hanlon JJ Picket GE. Ibid. 5.

3. Winslow CEA. The Untilled Fields of Public Health. Modern Medicine 1920; 2: 183.

4. Declaration of Joint UNICEF/WHO Conference. Alma Ata, Russia 1979: WPR/HMD/SPH/10/Inf 14-15.

5. Gershenson CP. Child Maltreatment, Family Stress, and Ecological Insult. Am.J. Public Health 1977; 67:602.

6. Taylor CE. Health Services in Developing Countries. In: Maxcy-Rosenau Public Health nd Preventive Medicine. 11th ed. New York 1980: Appleton-Crofts: 1701.

7. In Brief: The Johns Hopkins School of Hygiene and Public Health. 1983: 9.

Chapter I

HEALTH IN THE DEVELOPING WORLD

The aims of this chapter are twofold: a) to discuss common features of health in developing countries as an introduction to health in Saudi Arabia, and b) to argue that as long as there are differences between developed and developing countries in health problems, resources and population structure, the strategy for health development has to be different. With the pressing challenge to achieve health for all by the year 2000, the authorities in the developing countries must think rationally and innovatively for themselves.

The World Health Situation

The health situation in many developing countries gives a feeling of sadness and frustration. The warning message given by the General Director of the World Health Organization (WHO) on the health situation of the world (1981) is quite alarming[1].

-   Four-fifths of the world's population have no permanent form of health care.

-   The threat posed by such major diseases as malaria, schistosomiasis, filariasis, tryponosomiasis, leishmaniasis, cholera, and leprosy either has not lessened in recent years or has actually increased. Almost a quarter of the world's population remains infested with worms.

- Only one in three persons in developing countries has reasonable access to safe water and adequate sanitation.

- Infant mortality rates remain high in all developing countries and the rate of improvement has begun to slacken.

- More than five million children defecate themselves to death annually.

- More than half of all child deaths can be traced to the vicious complex of malnutrition, diarrhea and respiratory diseases. All of these deaths are unnecessary.

- A newborn child in some African countries has only a 50/50 chance of surviving through adolescence.

In his report on the State of the World's Children 1981-1982, the Executive Director of the United Nations Childrens Fund (UNICEF) stated that "the optimism of the 1960's which gave ground to the realism of the 1970's has now receded even further to make room for the doubt and pessimism which seems to be setting into the 1980's."[2] He provided us with some statistics as well.

- 17 million children died before their fifth birthday during 1981. They were simply failed by the world into which they were born.

- Not 10 percent of these children were immunized against the six most common and dangerous diseases of childhood.

- Less than US$ 100, if wisely spent on each of the poorest 500 million mothers and young children in the world could have bought improved diets and easier pregnancies, elementary education, basic health care, safer sanitation and more water. In other words, it could have bought the basics of life.

The director of the "Health for All" program in WHO estimates that fewer people have access to primary health care now than five years ago, except in certain countries and certain parts of these countries.[3]

Lack of rationale is a global phenomenon. The world spends about US$ 600 billion per year on the arms race (more than US$ 1,000,000 per minute), whereas more than 600 million people in the developing countries are not getting enough to eat. The world stockpile of nuclear weapons is equal to 16 billion tons of dynamite (3.6 tons per individual). Ninety-six percent of the nuclear weapons stockpile is kept in the USA and the USSR, yet both countries together have only 11 percent of the world's population.[4] In World War II only 3,000,000 tons of ammunition was exploded and 45 million people were killed. How many will be left alive after World War III?

The reasons behind the "unhealthy" present situation are mainly lack of finance, ineffective management, irrational use of resources and inappropriate training of health manpower.

Differences Between Developed and Developing Countries

Economically speaking the world population could be divided into least developing countries, developing countries and developed countries. There are differences between these countries in health and related socioeconomic indicators as the following statistic show (Tables 1, 2, 3, 4 and Figure 1).

Table 1. Health and Related Socioeconomic Indicators.

Index	Least Developed Countries	Other Developing Countries	Developed Countries
Number of countries	31	89	37
Total Population (Millions)	283	3,001	1,131
Infant Mortality Rate (per 1,000 live births)	160	94	19
Life Expectancy (Years)	45	60	72
Infants with birth weight of 2,500 g. or more (%)	70 %	83 %	93 %
Population with access to safe water supply (%)	31 %	41 %	100 %
Adult Literacy Rate	28 %	55 %	98 %
GNP per capita (US $)	170	520	6,230
Per capita public expenditure on health (US.$)	1.7	6.5	244
Public expenditure on health as %of GNP	1 %	1.2%	3.9%
Population per doctor	17,000	2,700	500
Population per nurse	6,500	1,500	220
Population per healthworker (any type including traditional birth attendant)	2,400	500	130

Source: WHO Chron/June 1981 35:223.

Table 2. Infant Mortality Per 1,000 Live Births in Selected Countries (1978 - 1980).

Afghanistan	169.0
Mali	120.0
Egypt	85.0
Barbados	22.0
Finland	7.7
Japan	7.5

Source: World Health Statistical Annual, WHO, Geneva 1982.

Table 3. Age Specific Death Rate 1––5 Years Per 1,000 Population in Selected Regions (1975).

Sub-Sahara (Africa)	>30.
Northern Africa	30.
Asia	>10.
Latin America	6.
Developed Regions	0.4 - 2.0

Source: World Health Forum 1981; 2 (2): 264.

Table 4. Aging In Selected Countries.

Country	Year	Total Pop. (Million)	65+ Years (Million)	Percent
Yugoslavia	1978	22.	2.1	10
U.K.	1980	49.2	7.4	15
Sweden	1980	8.3	1.4	17
Italy	1980	57.1	7.4	13
Germany	1980	62.	9.6	15
Poland	1980	36.	3.6	10
Greece	1979	9.5	1.2	12
Turkey	1975	40.	1.9	5
India	1980	664.	23.0	4
Japan	1980	117.	10.7	9

Source: U.N. Demographic Yearbook 1981.

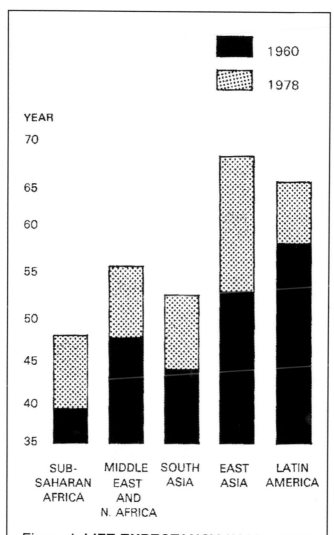

Figure 1. **LIFE EXPECTANCY (1960 - 1978)**

In developing countries, infectious diseases, malnutrition and inadequate environmental sanitation, as well as illiteracy and poverty, are the main factors behind high morbidity and mortality. In developed countries the causes are mostly metabolic and degenerative diseases (diseases of affl ue nee).

In developing countries the burden of diseases and death falls on young children; up to 50 percent of all deaths occur in children under five years of age while in the United States, 7 percent of all deaths occur in this age group. The chances of death before reaching puberty is 1 to 4 in many developing countries, while in developed countries it is 1 to 40. Table 5 shows the major causes of death in the under five years of age category in four developing countries.[5]

Table 5. Major Causes of Deaths Among 0-5 Years Age Group (Percentage).

Diseases	Imesi Nigeria	Luapula Zambia	North Sumatra	Pusan South Korea
	(1957)	(1972)	(1975)	(1956)
Diarrheal Diseases	12	18	25	15
Pneumonia	12	10	11	9
Protein-Calorie Malnutrition	12	16	26	14
Malaria	8	15	8	3
Pertussis	8	—	2	4
Measles	8	13	7	16
Tuberculosis	5	—	6	8
Smallpox	5	—	—	—
Anemia	—	7	5	—
Other Conditions (Mostly neonatal)	30	21	10	24

The problem with developing countries is not always the lack of resources but rather the failure to apply basic available knowledge in the proper way. It has been estimated that if all the knowledge of medicine and public health already available by the 1960's had been effectively applied including environmental measures, immunization, epidemiological control, early diagnosis and treatment and nutritional programs, most causes of morbidity could have been controlled or even eradicated (Table 6).[6]

Table 6. Possible Reduction in Deaths, by Cause, If All the Knowledge Available by 1960's had been Used.

Cause of Death	Reduction%
Typhoid and Paratyphoid	100
Meningococcal Infection	100
Streptococcal Infection	100
Pertussis	100
Diphtheria	100
Tuberculosis - all forms	100
Dysenteries	100
Malaria	100
Syphilis	100
Measles	100
Poliomyelitis	100
Neoplasms	50
Premature Births	70
Accidents	50

Determinants of Health

Ethnicity

Some ethnic groups are more susceptible to certain diseases than others. Several examples could be cited. Hypertension and active pulmonary tuberculosis are more common among black Americans than white Americans. The most common malignancies in white Europeans are those of the lungs, breast, stomach and colon, while in black Africans the predominant cancers are those of the skin, penis, cervix and liver. Chronic lymphatic leukemias are common among Jews but uncommon among Japanese and Chinese. The European races are said to be more susceptable to yellow fever than are native races of West Africa. Thalassaemias occur predominantly in people from the Mediterranean and Southeast Asia.

These differences could be explained by a combination of racial and genetic constitutions (intrinsic), and environmental (extrinsic) factors. It is difficult in most cases to distinguish between the relative roles of nature and nurture. Environment, however, plays the major role in most of the diseases.

Environment

Man is part of a micro environment (his habitat) and a macro environment (the universe around him). Environment, plays the major role in determining the health status of a population. It is a combination of social, physical and biological factors (Fig. 2). Poverty, illiteracy, overcrowding, unsafe water supply, unsanitary excreta disposal and contaminated water all may lead to an adverse effect on man's health.

History has taught us that environmental factors are the main determinants of health. The improvement of man's health in the modern ages is the result of sanitary developments and social reform more than anything else, including the advancement of medical technology.

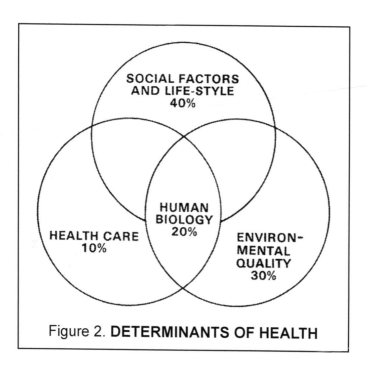

Figure 2. **DETERMINANTS OF HEALTH**

In the Middle Ages (AD 500 to 1500), Europe was passing through a period of scientific somnolence. The people were living in a low standard of housing, sanitation and personal hygiene. During the 1340's, the black death (bubonic plague) swept throughout the world. The total mortality is thought to have been over 60 million. Europe was almost devastated; in many places in France only two out of 20 survived. The disease destroyed half of the population of medieval England and at least 100,000 in London alone.[7]

The decline of morbidity in Europe had started well before the discovery of the actual cause of infectious diseases, or even the invention of specific treatments. This could be illustrated by the decline of tuberculosis in England and Wales. (Figure 3.)

In 1849 the mortality rate from cholera in England and Wales was 300 per 100,000 population, and it was vanishing by the end of the 19th century before the discovery of the organism by Koch in 1883 or the introduction of chemotherapy and rehydration techniques. The sharp decline of deaths from measles in Britain by the early 1900's was earlier than the application of measles vaccine.[8] (Figure 4.)

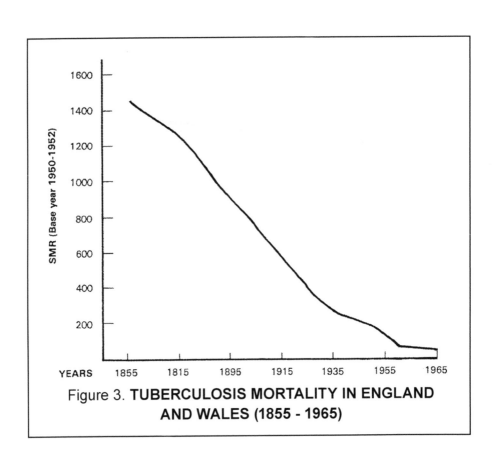

Figure 3. **TUBERCULOSIS MORTALITY IN ENGLAND AND WALES (1855 - 1965)**

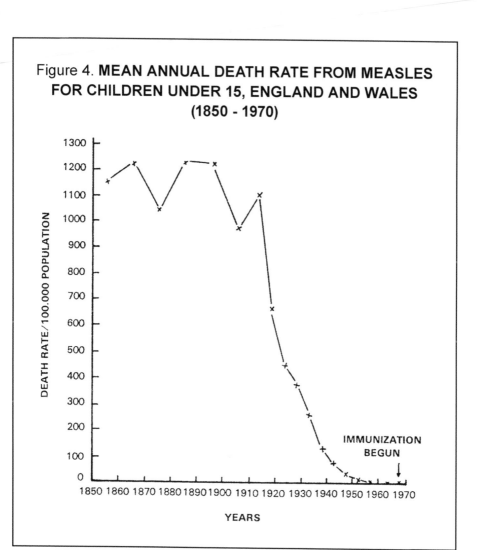

Figure 4. **MEAN ANNUAL DEATH RATE FROM MEASLES FOR CHILDREN UNDER 15, ENGLAND AND WALES (1850 - 1970)**

Over the centuries the life expectancy at birth has changed tremendously. In the 17th century only 50 percent of the population survived to their 15th birthday. In the 19th century and in 1970, 50 percent survived until the age of 40 and the age of 70 respectively.[9]

The United States of America has been subjected to a variety of scourges and epidemics in the past. Yellow fever was epidemic in the United States during the 18th and 19th centuries and malaria was endemic in the southern states until the 1940s. Health indices in the United States of America have changed a great deal over time. (Table 7.)

Table 7. Change in Health Indices in the USA by the Time (1900 - 1980).

	1900	1980
Infant Mortality Rate/1,000 Live Births	200.0	11.7
1 –– 5 Year Death Rate/1,000 Population	22.0	0.6
Life Expectancy at Birth	49.0	74.0

Source: World Health Statistical Annual, WHO, Geneva 1982.

Comparative health studies also give evidence that environmental factors, more than racial constitutions, create the difference in health among populations. Gordon[10] found that Japanese men living in the United States have a lower mortality rate from heart disease than white Americans. Japanese living in Japan have a much lower rate and those living in Hawaii are between these extremes. In our study in Turaba[11] we found that the weight of Turaba children below three months of age is slightly lower than Boston children of the same age group. The difference, however, becomes significant later in childhood due to environmental influences.

Measurements of children's growth has shown that until they reach five years of age, children in nearly all populations have the potential to grow as tall as

American children. This means that children in less developed countries are short, mostly because of poor nutrition.[12]

A village on the Nile Delta was surveyed in 1935 and 1979 for schistosomiasis using the same technique. During the 44 year period, a change in the pattern of prevalence was observed. Schistosoma mansoni infection increased from 3.2 percent to 73 percent and schistosoma hematobium infection decreased from 74 percent to 2.2 percent. The change has been attributed to a change in the ecosystem after the construction of the Aswan High Dam.[13]

Economic Status

Economic status is one of the most important factors affecting health both directly and indirectly; directly in terms of health resources (personnel, drugs, hospital beds, etc.) and indirectly through housing, nutrition, education, transportation, etc. To a great extent the effect of economy depends on how much it could possibly change the life style of the people.

The economic status of people is usually defined in terms of GNP, per capita GNP and per capita income. The disadvantage of these definitions is that they usually fail to express utilization and distribution. Nevertheless they are helpful measures.

Table 8 gives an example of GNP* per capita of selected countries and the number of years needed to achieve the 1965 US GNP per capita.

---

* **GNP: Gross National Product** The market value of all the goods and services produced in a nations economy. The World Bank defines countries with 1980 GNP of US$410 and below, as low income.

Table 8. GNP Per Capita of Selected Countries.

Country	GNP Per Capita 1965 (US $)	No. of Years Needed To Reach 1965 US GNP Per Capita (3,600)
Indonesia	99	593
Columbia	277	358
Nigeria	83	162
Mexico	455	162
Pakistan	91	144
France	1924	18
East Germany	1574	17
West Germany	1905	16
Canada	2464	12
Sweden	2497	11

Source. J. Bryan, Health in Developing World. Cornell University Press 1969:28.

The World Bank reported in 1979 that the total number of people living in absolute poverty was 780 million and the number would fall to 720 million by the end of 1980. Unfortunately that figure grew to 800 million.

The richest 20 percent of the world population has 71 percent of the world's products, while the poorest 20 percent has 2 percent of the world's products. In the 24 rich countries, food consumption averages 30 to 50 percent above requirements, and in the least developed countries the average consumption is 10 to 30 percent below requirements.

"In absolute terms, the north/south income gap is steadily widening. Income per capita now exceeds $8,600 a year in developed countries, but it is below $750 a year in the 34 poorest countries of the world."[14]

The gap will be further widened as a result of differences in population growth and GNP per capita growth rates. (Figure 5)

This uneven distribution of resources is expected and to some extent it is a natural phenomenon. In many instances, however, the scarcely available resources are not optimally utilized. This is either due to political instability, inefficient management, deficient planning, brain-drain of human resources, or a combination of all. The problem could be partially solved if developing countries have the will and the political commitment to chose the right approach. The least developed countries still would need technical and financial assistance from more developed countries.

Life Style

Life style is determined by a combination of physical factors and ethics, values, habits and customs. It has the greatest effect of all predisposing conditions on health.

In Saudi Arabia, for example, obesity, diabetes, hypertension, mental and emotional stress and road injuries became major causes of morbidity in big cities in the last two decades. Apparently it is due to the sudden changes in life style as a result of economic development, urbanization and competitive life. The Bedouin mother is shifting from breastfeeding her baby to the bottle - a symbol of modernization - with a possible increase of infantile diarrhea.[15] Dental caries is a major problem in Bisha because of a high consumption of dates and lack of oral hygiene.[16] Schistosomiasis in Baha is a recreational disease. It affects school children while swimming in the Wadis (waterbeds) infested with snails.[17] Trachoma in Qasim affects 92 percent of children because of lack of personal hygiene.[18]

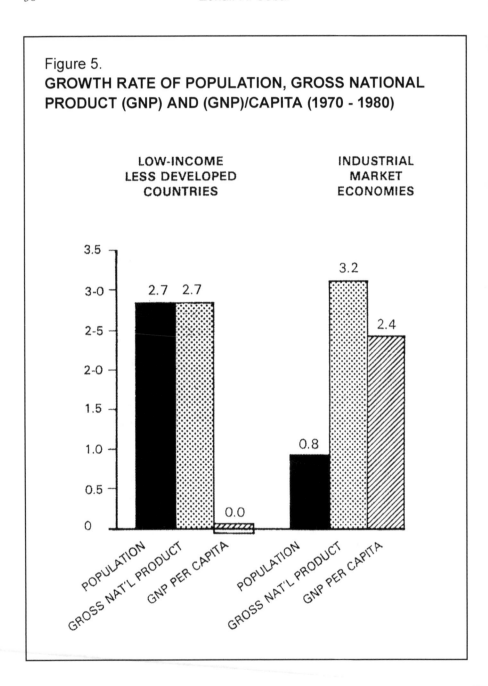

Figure 5.
GROWTH RATE OF POPULATION, GROSS NATIONAL
PRODUCT (GNP) AND (GNP)/CAPITA (1970 - 1980)

A study carried out in rural and urban areas of South Lebanon found that educated women and women living in urban areas were better off in terms of family formation patterns, immunization and well-baby care.[19]

In Egypt, the villagers keep their animals under their roofs because animals are precious and dear to them. A villager prefers to drink directly from the Nile river rather than from piped clean water; the Nile gives fertility to the land and will give him, he believes, fertility as well.

The higher rate of cardiovascular disease in the world is found in North Karelia, Finland. The predominant risk factor is the high cholesterol diet of the townspeople.[20]

In order to improve the health situation in a community, health programs should be directed to improving the behavior of the people as well as to manipulating the physical environment. To change human behavior, however, requires a change in knowledge, attitude and practice, which is quite a challenge.

Nutrition

Nutritional problems are a consequence of poverty and life-style. Malnutrition results from insufficient consumption, absorption or utilization of food. It can be due to problems of food supply, food accessibility, dieting patterns (taste, tradition and perception) and distribution between and within families.

During infancy, especially in the neonatal period, the child's health reflects the mother's nutritional status. Low birth weight, iron deficiency, anemia and beriberi, for example, are common problems of infants born to malnourished mothers. During the postnatal period, bottle feeding practice and poor weaning habits aggravated by unhygienic conditions and lack of immunization can lead to synergetic effect of malnutrition, diarrhea and pneumonia, the triad responsible for the high rate of infant morbidity and mortality in developing countries. Undernourished infants have low disease resistance which may cause them to die from what would be minor diseases under better circumstances (measles case mortality in Guatemala in 1976, for instance, was 268 times that in the U.S.).[21] At the extreme end of the protein calorie deficiency we find kwashirkor and marasmus. Chronic malnutrition may lead to stunted physical development, impaired cognitive abilities, low performance in school, susceptibility to infectious diseases and low economic productivity.

Population Dynamics

Natural population growth is the difference between birth and death rates. From early recorded history, population growth was sustained at a low pace; the high birth rate was always balanced by a high death rate. By the end of the 17th century, death rates started to slow down with a progressive increase in the population growth (Table 9). By the midddle of the 19th century a difference in population growth started to show between economically developed countries and less developed countries as a result of social reforms and the progression in science and technology. (Table 10).

Table 9. Estimated World Population 8000 BC to AD 1970 with Projection to AD 2,000, Annual Rates of Increase and Years to Double.

Year	Estimated Population (Millions)	Annual Rate of Increase In Preceding Interval (%)	Years for Population To Double at Given Rate of Increase
8000 BC	10	--	--
0	250	0.04	1,730
1650 AD	470	0.04	1,730
1850	1,240	0.5	139
1950	2,485	0.7	99
1970	3,632	1.9	37
1980	4,457	2.1	33
2000	6,494	1.9	37

Source: United Nations Population Studies; No. 48, 1970. Data derived from Hauser, Science 131:1641, 1960, also from various United Nations surveys; 50, 53, 54.

Table 10. Demographic Patterns in Developing and Developed Regions of the World.

	Developing Regions	Developed Regions
Live Birth Rate/1000 Pop.	45	18
Crude Death Rate/1000 Pop.	20	10
% Population Increase/Year	2.5	0.8
Years Needed to Double Population	25	80
% of Population Under 1 5 years	40	20
% of Population Over 65 Years	6	11
% of People Living in Rural Areas	80	20

Many economists argue that the current accelerated population growth will have a negative impact on the socioeconomic and welfares situation in developing countries. In their view it will absorb any marginal improvement in gross national products, leaving nothing for prosperity or development and even add to the distress.

Many problems are considered to be linked to the uncontrolled population growth including rapid urbanization and its by-products of slums, violence, delinquencies and environmental pollution. The United Nations estimates that between 1980 and 2000 the capital cities of Bangladesh and Zambia may triple in size; Lagos and Nairobi may almost quadruple.

The expected high ratio of young economically unproductive population adds another burden on the poor economy. This is usually accompanied by a high rate of unemployment and underemployment among adults (up to 40 percent in some developing countries).

Most experts on the problem either hold, on technological grounds, that the earth can adequately support several times its present population, or warn, on ecological grounds, that the earth is already overpopulated and that human numbers should be reduced. A third group holds the view that the world is not yet overpopulated but will be so in the second decade of the 21st century.[22]

Robert McNamara, the former President of the World Bank, is very pessimistic in his statement, "Short of thermonuclear war itself, population growth is the gravest issue the world faces over the decades immediately ahead."[23] There is, however, a ray of optimism. Theoretically the photosynthesis process at its maximum efficiency uses 8 percent of sunlight. This is sufficient to feed three million million people, i.e. 900 times the present million population. However, this number of population, if achieved 350 years from today will give each individual an area of only 10 x 16 meters of space!

From these arguments one might conclude that the problem is rather an irrational utilization of resources. While more than half of the world population lives in undernourished areas and more than 800 million people live in absolute poverty, the world spends $600 billion every year on the arms race, and rich countries destroy tons of agricultural products to keep market prices high.

In Egypt, most of the 44 million population lives on 4 percent of the land strip surrounding the Nile River. Sudan's crop land alone could supply the Arab world with much of its needs in agricultural products if better utilized. Less than 5 percent of its fertile land is being utilized.

Which Way Forward?

Statistics show us that most of the world population is deprived of basic health services. In many developing countries less than US$5 is being spent on health per capita per year; the 25 poorest countries in the world spend an average of US$2.6 per person per year.

In general, the present approach to health development is fragmented and irrational. A recent WHO survey carried out in 70 out of 134 countries which signed the Alma Ata Decree, showed that most of them find it difficult to live up to their commitment.[24]

Let us, as a reminder, go back to the warning message of the General Director of WHO on the health situation in the world in the year 1981.

- Four-fifths of the world's population have no permanent form of health care.

- The threat posed by major diseases has either not lessened in recent years or has actually increased. Almost a quarter of the world's population remain infested with worms.

- Only one in three persons in developing countries has reasonable access to safe water and adequate sanitation.

With such a gloomy picture one wonders what magic could change the situation in the next 17 years in order to achieve the goal "health for all by the year 2000."

Is the economy of the world going to improve and will more money be available to the health sector?

Is the political commitment of the 134 member states of WHO which signed the Alma Ata Decree going to be fulfilled so that health will be considered as an objective of economic development?

Are health authorities and medical educators going to change their attitudes from individual patient care to the holistic approach to health?

How can the dream be turned into a reality?

Three features of health are predominant in the developing world:

1. The health problems are largely determined by socioeconomic and environmental factors rather than by genetic, racial or built-in errors of metabolism.

2. Health resources are limited because of absolute or relative poverty.

3. The already limited resources are not optimally utilized. More emphasis is usually given to glorious and prestigious projects rather than those that are needed.

What is the cure, or rather, the prevention of this dilemma? Suggestions for improvement could be summarized as follows:

Holistic Approach

Health educators, planners, decision-makers and executives should adopt a holistic approach to health, considering health development as an end and a means which has to be integrated with socioeconomic development. The Director General of WHO, in defining the meaning of "health for all by the year 2000," stressed that "health, social awareness and socioeconomic development should go hand in hand, the one leading and reinforcing the other." He cited an example: by controlling one parasite in a rural African village, the cultural output could improve.[25] A sick person cannot be economically productive and ill health is a mechanism of perpetuating the cycle of poverty. Optimum health status can only be achieved by protecting people from being sick in the first place and by treating the sick. This holistic approach could be accomplished by:

a. Comprehensive health care - preventive, promotive and curative.

b. Coordination between the Ministries of Health and other related sectors, governmental and non-governmental.

c. Coordination between medical education institutions and health services sectors.

d. Community participation.

Improvement of Medical Education.

A long list of suggestions could be made on how to improve the health status of the people in developing countries. The one simple suggestion on top of the list would be to "improve medical education."

Medical education involves education of all the members of the health team. Physicians, in their capacities as decision makers, planners and medical educators, need a special concern. All over the world the majority of physicians have received, or are still receiving, their training in curative-oriented and hospital-based medical schools. They mostly tend to view the solution of the problem from one end of the spectrum - the treatment of the patient - instead of the whole spectrum of treatment and prevention.

During the hearing of a three-year study appraising medical education in the United States and Canada, the following observations were made:[26]

"Medical students (and therefore doctors) are usually not well educated persons in the broadest sense."

"Students get their tickets punched in the humanities, without the reflection and insight into the human condition which are the expected outcome of such exposure".

The study continues by stating "Both medical school faculty and students are facing a dilemma caused by the explosion of new knowledge and technology. Students are expected to be independent learners with analytic and problem-solving skills but are trained in a system dominated by teaching and examination methods that often do not promote those techniques. They are being taught by faculty members who should be serving as guides to assist students rather than as conveyors of information that is available in books, journals and other media."

As a response to these statements, an 18-member panel, chaired by the president of Johns Hopkins University, has a goal to formulate suggestions that will make a sound medical education system better in preparing physicians who are skilled professionals and humanists as well.

This is in the United States and Canada. What would be the findings of a study conducted in the developing world?

In his article "Medical Technology in Developing Countries, Useful, Useless, or Harmful?" McCord argues that "In many of the developing countries, the professional groups relate more to the needs of an industrialized society than to those of their own nation. It is not at all an exaggeration to say that the need is for appropriate people, not an appropriate technology."[27]

A physician should be trained to maintain good health for his people and curative care is one aspect in the process. To achieve his objective, the physician should assume the role of educator, coordinator, planner and promoter as well as medical practitioner.

The great physicians of the past were philosophers, astronomers, historians, social reformers and spiritual leaders. The modern physician, regardless of his specialty, can still be a man of vision.

It is self evident that the five to seven years of medical education curriculum is not enough to cover all the knowledge of medical and clinical sciences, putting aside humanities and behavioral sciences. The only way is to provide medical students with the basic knowledge and skills, the right attitude and the ability of self learning. This is the biggest challenge in designing a medical education curriculum.

Continuing Education

Development of available and potential human resources through continuing education programs should receive the utmost attention. The goals are:

a.   to improve awareness and common understanding of the comprehensive health care concept, objectives and methodologies;

b.   to create willingness and commitments; and

c.   to improve skills of planning and implementation.

Continuing education programs include reorientation courses, seminars, conferences, workshops, study tours, etc. It should cover all the members of the health team especially the following categories:

a. Policy Makers.

Policy makers in sectors such as finance, planning, education, social welfare and municipalities should be oriented toward their responsibilities in health development. The meeting held in Tehran in 1978 on Health Services and Health Manpower Development is a good example of how a common language could be developed in a convention.[28] Among the participants were top planners and executives from the ministries of health, education and social welfare as well as medical educators from Middle East countries.

b. Health Authorities and Educators.

There is an immense need to enhance the capabilities of many health authorities and educators in planning and implementing national health programs. Refresher courses should be designed for them in the areas of management, economy, budgeting, planning, programming, policital science, human behavior, population dynamics and demography.

c. Practicing Physicians.

Many practicing physicians function as policy makers, planners and directors of the health services. They should be prepared to undertake such a comprehensive role.

d. Training of the Health Team.

In many countries emphasis lies on the training of physicians rather than all members of the health team (physicians, nurses, sanitarians, health visitors, health educators and others). This leads to an inverted health manpower pyramid and unproductive system. It is well documented that health auxilliaries can have great impact in improving the health of the people, if well trained and directed. The Kavar Village Health Worker Project was a pilot project in southern Iran designed to test the effectiveness of rural health auxilliaries. Results showed that auxilliaries have drastically reduced both infant mortality and overall mortality.[29] In another project in western Azerbaijan, Iran, the delivery of environmental and primary health care services by indigenous front-line health workers (FLHW) resulted in a significant decline in crude birth and death rates and in infant and one-to-five year mortality rates.[30] A survey among Iranian villages indicates that they are far more likely to prefer Iranian auxilliaries than non-Iranian physicians.[31]

Community Participation

People can be a tremendous resource if they are prepared to take a positive and responsible role in the health system. Without the understanding and participation of the public many programs would fail. In Western Azerbijan, Iran, the community, with the initiative of the health assistant, carried the expenses of establishing a piped water system, paved roads and public latrines.

Both health needs and demands should be considered. Health needs are what the experts think are necessary, such as environmental sanitation, immunization programs and prenatal care. Health demands are what people think necessary such as hospitals, injections, x-ray machines, etc. In developing countries where people are, by and large, illiterate and uninformed, the gap between health needs and demands is wide. (Figure 6.)

Developing of Primary Health Care.

The International Conference on Primary Health Care, held at Alma Ata, Russia in 1978, expressed the need for urgent action by all governments, all health and development workers, and the world community to protect the health of the people of the world.[32] The declaration of the meeting stated that "A main social target of governments, international organizations and the whole world community should be the attainment by all the people of the world, by the year 2000, of a level of health that will permit them to lead a socially and economically productive life. Primary care is the key to this target."

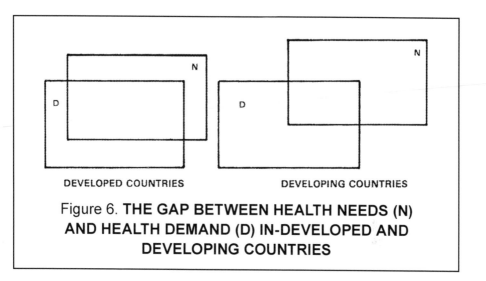

DEVELOPED COUNTRIES   DEVELOPING COUNTRIES

Figure 6. **THE GAP BETWEEN HEALTH NEEDS (N) AND HEALTH DEMAND (D) IN-DEVELOPED AND DEVELOPING COUNTRIES**

The declaration went on to define primary health care as:

a. essential health care based on practical, scientifically sound and socially acceptable methods.

b. a solution to the main health problems in the community through promotive, preventive, curative and rehabilitative services.

c. including health education, promotion of food supply and proper nutrition, adequate supply of safe water and basic sanitation, maternal and child health care, prevention and control of common diseases and injuries.

Primary health care, especially in the developing world, can meet more than 80 percent of the health needs of the people, as long as it provides comprehensive care (promotive, preventive and curative). At the present time, health care provided by health centers, sub-centers, health points and traditional healers throughout the world, is predominantly curative or even palliative in nature.

Some countries have started primary health care projects with a comprehensive health care approach. Among these projects are Rizaia Project in Iran, Karaiba Experimental Project in Sudan, Loiza Primary Health Care Center in Puerto

Rico, the integrated child development service scheme in India, the Pikine Project in Senegal, the Lampang Health Development Project in Thailand and the Solo Project in Indonesia. Most of these projects, years after their establishment, still remain experimental. They were started as vertical programs, lacking the means to expand and become integrated in the health systems.

A new specialty, Family Medicine, emerged in North America and Western Europe in the late 1960s and other countries have followed the trend. In 1983 the author had a chance to attend the Tenth World Conference on Family Medicine in Singapore, organized by WONCA (The World Organization of National Colleges, Academics and Academic Association of General Practitioners and Family Practitioners). Several hundred participants from all over the world attended. A striking feature was that the conference was influenced throughout by the western style of family medicine, i.e. patient care rather than comprehensive approach.

It was a warning sign that developing countries might copy a style which does not necessarily fit their needs.

Conclusion

With such differences between developed and developing countries in economic status, cultural pattern, health ecology and rates of morbidity and mortality, the medical care system has to be different. It requires maximum utilization of scarce resources (manpower, money and management) in order to obtain optimum health. Such a system should emphasize:

-   Relevant medical education

-   Continuing education and self-learning

-   Rational planning

-   Comprehensive health care (curative, preventive and promotive)

- Team work

- Community participation

- Appropriate technology

BIBLIOGRAPHY

1. Mahler H. The meaning of "Health for All by the Year 2000" World Health Forum 1981; 2(1): 5-22.

2. Grant J P. "The State of the World's Children 1981-1982". Report to UNICEF 1982: 13.

3. World Health Magazine, Sept. 1983.

4. Sward R. World Military and Social Expenditure. World Priority 1982.

5. Morley D. Paediatric Priorities in the Developing World, London: Butterworths & Co., 1973:318.

6. Halon JJ. Principles of Public Health Administration, Saint Louis: The C.V. Mosby Company, 1964:97.

7. Halon JJ. ibid. 1984: 25; From: Hecker IF. The Epidemics of the Middle Ages. Philadelphia: Haswell, Barrington and Haswell, 1837.

8. Basch PF. International Health, New York: Oxford University, 1978:94.

9. Lowe CR Health Needs and Health Services: A Question of Priorities. The Central African Journal of Medicine 1975: 229-35.

10. Gordon T. Mortality Experience Among the Japanese in the United States, Hawaii and Japan. Public Health Report 1957; Vol. No. 6(72): 543-53.

11. Sebai ZA. The Health of the Family in a Changing Arabia. 3rd ed. Jeddah: Tihama, 1983: 85.

12. Nutrition. AID Policy Paper, US Agency for International Development: Washington D.C. 20523, May 1982: ii.

13. Abdel-Wahab MF, et al. Chaning Pattern of Schistosomiasis in Egypt 1935-79. Lancet 1979 August 4: 242-4.

14. Population Crisis Committee. World Population Growth and Global Security. Population Sept. 1983; 13:5.

15. Sebai ZA. The Health of the Family in a Changing Arabia. 3rd ed. Jeddah: Tihama, 1983: 114.

16. Sebai ZA. Dental Health in Bisha Town. Unpublished Report to Ministry of Health, 1978.

17. Alio IS. Epidemiology of Schistosomiasis in Saudi Arabia with Emphasis on Geographic Distribution Pattern. ARAMCO, Dhahran, 1967.

18. Badr I, Qureshi I. Ocular Status of School Children in Al Asiah - Qasim Region. In: Sebai ZA, ed. Community Health in Saudi Arabia. Saudi Medical Journal Monograph No. 1. Riyadh 1982: 26.

19. Zurayk H, et al. Effect of Urban Versus Rural Residents and of Maternal Education on Infant Health in South Lebanon. Journal of Epidemiology and Community Health, 1982; 36: 192-6.

20. Klein SD. Class, Culture and Health. In: Maxcy - Rosenau Public Health and Preventive Medicine. J.M. Last Ed. New York: Appleton-Crofts, 1980; 1028.

21. Nutrition. AID Policy Paper, US Agency for International Development: Washington D.C. 20523, May 1982:1.

22. Gilland B. Considerations on World Population and Food Supply. Population and Development Review June 1983; Vol. 9. No. 2: 203.

23. Population Crisis Committee. World Population Growth and Global Security. Population Sept. 1983; 13: 1.

24. Progress in Primary Health Care: A Situation Report. World Health Organization, 1983.

25. O'Mahoney V. et al. The Least Developed Countries: A Substantial New Programme of Action for the 1980's. WHO Chronicle 1981; 35: 225.

26. Hinz AC. Study to Improve Medical School's Methods. American Medical News, November 1983: 20.

27. McCord C. Medical Technology in Developing Countries: Useful, Useless, or Harmful? The American Journal of Clinical Nutrition, December 1978:2301:13.

28. An Integrated Approach to Health Services and Manpower Development. WHO/EMRO Techinical Publication, 1978; 1.

29. Zeighami B., et al. Stretching Health Manpower: The Rural Health Auxilliary. Canadian Journal of Public Health, 1977: 68; 378-81.

30. Baezegar MA., et al. Evaluation of Rural Primary Health Care Services in Iran: Report on Vital Statistics in West Azarbaijan. Am J Public Health, 1981 Vol. 71, No. 7.

31. Zeighami B., et al. Physician Importation - A Solution to Developing Countries' Rural Health Care Problems? Am J Public Health, 1978; 68; No. 8: 378-81.

32. Declaration of Alma Ata. Joint UNICEF/WHO Conference. Alma Ata, Russia, 1979: WPR/HMD/SPH/10/Inf 14-15.

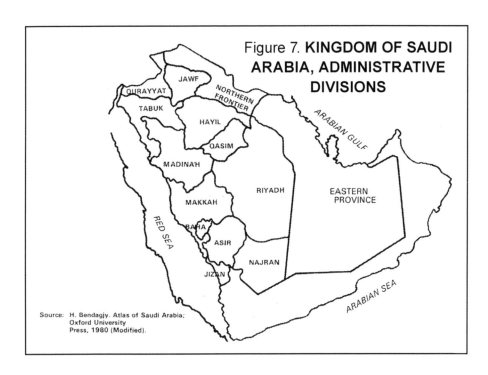

Figure 7. **KINGDOM OF SAUDI ARABIA, ADMINISTRATIVE DIVISIONS**

Source: H. Bendagjy. Atlas of Saudi Arabia; Oxford University Press, 1980 (Modified).

Chapter II

INTRODUCTION TO SAUDI ARABIA

"This Chapter presents a brief introduction to Saudi Arabia. Detailed information on the Country health problems, health manpower, health resources and population structure will be provided in Volume II."

GENERAL DEVELOPMENT

The Kingdom of Saudi Arabia occupies approximately four-fifths of the Arabian Peninsula, an area of 2,250,000 square kilometers. (Figure 7.)

The climate is hot and dry. A humid climate prevails along the coast for six months of the year. During the long summer months midday temperatures may reach 48°C. Winters are reasonably cool. The average annual rainfall throughout Arabia is generally very low, being five inches or less. Vegetation is sparse and widely scattered. The fauna is also limited. The most important crops are dates, wheat, barley, corn and alfalfa. Fruits and vegetables are being grown in increasing amounts.

Saudi Arabia is a monarchy whose constitution is the Koran and Sharia Law. The King heads the government and the Council of Ministers is the executive and administrative body.

In 1983 the population of Saudi Arabia was estimated at 9.7 million. The estimated ratio of Bedouins varies, the most widely accepted figure is less than 15 percent. Arabs, like Europeans, are largely of the Caucasian race. Bedouins are generally of the brown Mediterranean type. The population is predominantly Sunni Moslem mostly adhering to the Hanbali school of Islamic law. There is a minority of Shia, who live mainly in the Eastern Province.

Although the exploration for oil in the Eastern Province of Saudi Arabia began in early 1934, it was not drilled commercially until 1938. Suddenly, Saudi Arabia was catapulted into the 20th century. The traditional, isolated, poor and mostly Bedouin country began to modernize. For the past half century a progressive and persistent evolution has touched every aspect of life in Saudi Arabia. Culturally, socially and economically there have been changes, and more change is expected.

Saudi Arabia is economically stable and enjoys a strong foreign exchange position with a surplus balance of international payments. The government revenue increased from SR5.7 billion in 1970 to SR211 billion in 1980 (40 times). Oil revenue accounted for 90 percent of the total revenue. Table 1 shows some indices of progress in several fields during the period 1970 to 1980.

The per capita income is estimated at SR58,400 per annum, one of the highest in the world. The cost of living grew at an annual rate of 16.5 percent over the 1970 - 1980 period, a total increase of 350 percent.

Table 1. Indices of Progress in Saudi Arabia (1970 –– 1980).

Index	1970	1980
No. of Schools	3107	110,070
Students (Thousands)		
Primary and Intermediate	458	1,107
Secondary	16	93
University	7	48
Road Vehicles	60,000	2,000,000
Imported Cargo (Millions of Tons)	1.8	27.5
Paved Roads (Kilometers)	8,021	20,238

Source: Ministry of Planning, Saudi Arabia. Facts and Figure (1982).

Development in the public sector has focused on health, education, communications, agriculture, water resources, and mineral deposits.

In the private sector the effort has been to encourage private investment and to attract outside expertise for industrialization.

King Saud University, the first in the country, was established in 1957 with one college, the College of Arts. By 1984 there were seven universities with more than 40 colleges.

Health Services

The health services system, from the time of its organization in 195 0through the late 1960s, has developed slowly. However, during the last two decades, the country has experienced a rapid expansion of all aspects of socioeconomic life including the health services. The health problems in the Kingdom vary from communicable diseases, such as malaria and schistosomiasis, to those of a modern society with stress related diseases, pollution and an ever increasing number of road accidents. Vital statistics and data on morbidity and mortality and epidemiology of health problems are greatly deficient. The shortage of well-trained Saudi health personnel remains the principal difficulty.

The country is divided into 11 health regions each headed by a regional health director. Most of the planning and decision-making has been centralized in Riyadh, the capital. However, regionalization has started with more authority being delegated to the regional directors.

The history of organized preventive health services in Saudi Arabia began in the early 1950s when the Ministry of Health, ARAMCO and the World Health Organization launched the first campaign against malaria in Qatif and Hassa Oasis in the Eastern Province. Success led to a series of malaria control programs in central, western and southwestern Arabia. In the early 1980's the concept of primary health care became popular and the WHO slogan "health for all by the year 2000" became recognized.

The main objectives of health services in the Kingdom, as stated in the Third Development Plan (1400-1405/1980-1985) are:

-   Improvement of the health status of the people and the control of endemic diseases.

-   Providing all the people with free, comprehensive and integrated health services.

-   Improvement of health manpower.

-   Strengthening environmental health, preventive medicine and primary health care.

-   Encouragement of the private sector.

Table (2) shows development of health resources in the country over the 10 year period 1972 to 1982.

Table 2. Development of Health Services in Saudi Arabia.

	1972	1982
Hospitals	80	119
Beds	10,101	20,775
Health Centers	621	1,415
Physicians	1,704	9,799
Nurses	4,370	17,175
Health Assistants	2,230	9,484

Source: Ministry of Planning - Achievements of the Health Plan 1970 - 1982 (p. 163-165)

The average annual rates of growth for health manpower in the period 1972 to 1982 were 18.8 percent for physicians, 13.9 percent for nurses and 14.3 percent for health assistants. The increase in the total number of health personnel was 500 percent over the 10 year period.

The Ministry of Health provides 74 percent of hospital beds, 62 percent of physicians and 64 percent of nursing staff; the rest is provided by 15 other government organizations* and the private sector.

---

*   The main government agencies which provide health services are the Ministries of Defence and Aviation, Interior, Education, Municipalities, and Labour and Social Welfare, National Guard, Girls Education, Youth Department, Red Crescent and Universities.

In 1984 the Ministry of Health budget was SR10,742,000,000 (4.1 percent of the government's budget). This gives a per capita expenditure by the Ministry of Health only of SR 932 per year.

The expansion of the health services has depended primarily on expatriates from Arab countries, Europe, United States of America, the Indian subcontinent and the Far East. The recruitment of large numbers of expatriates has helped in extending the services to every town and village in the country. However, the diversity of educational and cultural backgrounds has presented problems, as has the uneven urban-rural distribution.

In order to increase the number of Saudi health personnel, four medical schools, a faculty of dentistry, a faculty of health sciences, a faculty of veterinary medicine, and a department of hospital administration were established between 1969 and 1980. The Faculty of Pharmacy was established in 1959.

There were 460 Saudi physicians in 1979 (9 percent of all physicians). By 1995 it is projected that there will be 4,450. They will be the product of the four medical schools in the country and of medical schools abroad. In spite of the expected improvement in the numbers of physicians there will still remain a shortage of other members of the health team.

In Saudi Arabia, the goals of reducing morbidity and mortality and of raising the standard of health among the people are easily attainable with appropriate planning and utilization of resources. What is encouraging is that the political will and commitment are there.

Chapter III

HEALTH PROFILE OF
SELECTED COMMUNITIES

This chapter discusses the health profile of selected rural communities in Saudi Arabia.

TURABA
KHULAIS
TAMNIA
QASIM

Turaba community was studied in 1967 as the field project for the author's degree in public health, and again in 1981 to observe any changes in the health services system. The other three communities, Khulais, Tamnia and Qasim were studied by teams of teachers and students from the Faculty of Medicine, King Saudi University, Riyadh, in the years 1977, 1979 and 1980 respectively. In this chapter the educational aspect of these studies, the methodology, and some of the epidemiological findings will be discussed.

The material presented here is excerpted from published books and articles which are referred to in the text. The findings, although reflecting a general health set up in rural Saudi Arabia, are not representative of the country.

I - TURABA
INTRODUCTION

This study of health indices and services in Turaba, Western Province of Saudi Arabia was conducted in two stages, in 1967 and 1981. It highlights the changes which have occurred over a period of 15 years in Turaba.*

In 1967, the author conducted the field research for his doctorate degree in public health in Turaba. Several years later, the author perceived that the primary care system in the country, as well as in many other developing countries he visited, does not fulfill its potential role in promoting the health of the people. In 1981, the author returned to Turaba for a short visit to observe development in the health services system and he noted little change in the quality of care.

In the author's opinion, the problem of primary health care in Saudi Arabia, as is the case in many other parts of the world, is related to the quality of personnel. In order to improve the primary health care system, the starting point would be to modify the primary focus of medical education, emphasizing a community-based, problem-solving approach.

Turaba is an area of approximately 18,500 square kilometers in west Saudi Arabia (Figure 8). There is no accurate census of the population of Turaba. It was estimated at 30,000 in 1967 and 45,000 in 1981.

Turaba could be divided into three communities:

A. Settled Community

The inhabitants live primarily in the two main towns of Souk and Alawa and have a history of settlement of more than 25 years. The main occupations are government employment, trade, and some

---

*   This section is an excerpt from the book "The Health of the Family in Changing Arabia."[1]

farming. In general they enjoy a better economy than the rest of the Turaba population and have ready access to the health center.

B. Semi-Settled Community

The inhabitants live mostly in settlement areas "hejrat" scattered along the two main wadis (water beds) and have a history of settlement of less than 25 years. Their economy depends on animal husbandry and some agriculture.

C. Nomadic Bedouins

The inhabitants are still nomads with no fixed residence. They wander seasonally from place to place within a defined territory. They live in tents and their main source of income is animal husbandry.

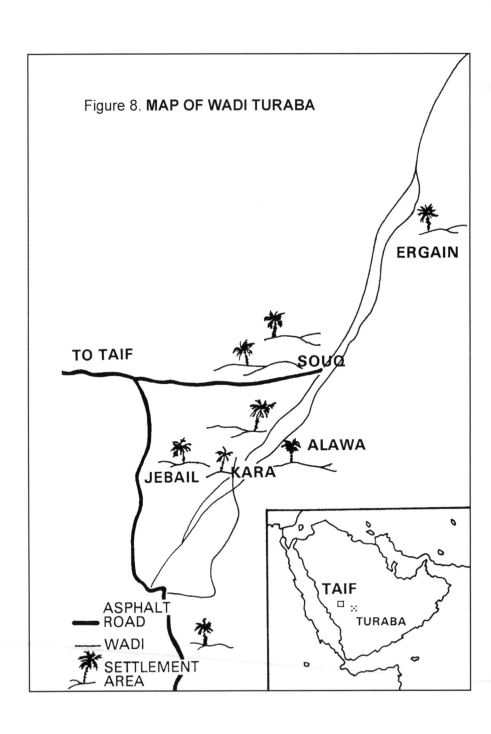

Figure 8. **MAP OF WADI TURABA**

77777777777777777

Souq, the oldest village, is the administrative capital and is located in the center of Turaba. It is connected by a 140 kilometer asphalt road to the city of Taif (approx. 250,000 population), the summer capital of the government.

The settlement of Bedouins has developed rapidly, mostly because of the drought and the improved economy of settled life. The estimated proportion of nomads decreased from 30 percent in 1967 to less than 20 percent in 1981.

According to a United Nations report, "the last nomadic Bedouin will pack his tent and migrate to the city by 1995."

Although the health center in Souq was expanded and its personnel increased during this period, its function did not change much; it still provides curative health services. This is not a unique situation. Studies in several communities in the country, Asir,[2] Hejaz,[3] and Qasim[4,5] as well as in other neighboring Arab countries[6,7] showed the same pattern. The problem looks crucial if we consider that these types of health centers provide primary health care for more than 70 percent of the population.

TURABA IN 1967

The Objectives

The objectives of the field survey conducted in 1967 were:

1. to determine the health status of children 0-4 years of age in selected settled, semi-settled and nomadic communities.

2. to identify the socioeconomic and environmental factors and available health services which might influence the children's health condition in each community.

The Methodology

Three hundred and fourteen households were selected in the three communities including 87 settled, 121 semi-settled and 106 nomadic households. Interviews, formal and informal, were held with the heads of the households and their wives to cover areas of demography, history of morbidity and mortality of children, nutrition, socioeconomic and environmental conditions, and health knowledge, attitudes and practices. Clinical, anthropometric and laboratory exminations were performed on children up to four years of age in the households under study.

A team of 18 persons, including social workers and laboratory assistants, worked from August to October of 1967 to collect the data required for the survey. The data was then transferred to the Johns Hopkins University School of Public Health, Baltimore, Maryland, for processing and analysis.

In presenting the findings, the three groups under study will be referred to as one community. Wherever there are significant differences among the three communities, each group will be referred to separately as:

Community A - Settled Community

Community 8 - Semi-settled Community

Community C - Nomadic Community

For further details of the methodology the reader is referred to the basis of this Chapter.

The Findings

Family Structure

The family in Turaba is a nuclear family with many children. The main reason for the change from the traditional extended family is the migration of the young adults and their families to the cities. The family is patriarchal. Cousin marriage in the paternal line is preferred. Male children are especially welcomed in the family. At the age of two, children are weaned. At the age of two to three years, boys are circumcised in elaborate ceremonies and at the age of seven years they are shifted to the man's world and enjoy the company of their fathers, while girls stay with their mothers. At that age, Bedouin boys and girls guard sheep under supervision.

Among the settled population, the average age of marriage for girls is 16 years. For Bedouin girls it is usually delayed until 18 because she is needed by her family for herding goats and sheep. In all three communities, marriage for girls might be as early as 13 or even younger.

By interviewing 332 mothers it was found that the average number of pregnancies per mother is 5.2. In the last year there were eight reported abortions. A woman is thought to have an abortion if she lifts a heavyweight, is beaten by her husband, or is affected by a supernatural power (will of God, touch of Jinn, Evil Eye). The touch of Jinn is believed to cause abortion as well as sterility, death of children, or the delay of childbirth for several years!

We did not dare ask, even in an informal way, about induced abortion. The only old Bedouin lady whom we asked about it became very angry, and her enraged reply was, "it is for prostitutes." Although induced abortion might be practiced occasionally, the religious feeling against it is very strong.

The woman is usually thought to be responsible for infertility and a man is considered responsible only in rare cases. The perceived causes of a man's sterility are smallpox and Jinn. The perceived causes of a woman's sterility are sickness, deformity or blockage of the womb, a Jinn taking the spermatozoa away, or if the woman steps over a grave.

Contrary to what is generally believed, polygamy is limited, particularly among nomads. We found the percentage of those who are married to more than one wife ranges between 5 percent in the nomadic community and 18 percent in the villages. There is a positive correlation between multiple marriages and the socioeconomic status. Among the younger generation in Saudi Arabia, however, polygamy is considered a stigma.

Divorce and remarriage is more frequent among nomads than among the settled and semi-settled people. Family ties do not appear to be affected by divorce in the nomadic community as much as in the settled community.

Knowledge, attitude and practice of family planning were critical subjects to ask about. When we started to ask mothers, "How many children would you like to have?" and "How can a woman prevent pregnancy?" we faced difficulties. The conservative community in Turaba did not accept this type of questions. Rumors arose that we were asking about the sexual relationship between a woman and her husband.

A total of 266 mothers answered the question "How many children do you want to have?" 23 percent said that they wanted more children, 23 percent said that they wanted no more children and the remaining 54 percent were indifferent, their answers being, "As God wishes," "I want health," or "I don't know." No significant difference was found between the three communities in their answers. One mother said: "I want as many children as the papers in your hand." Another one wanted five boys and one girl: "The boys will take care of me, but the girl will take of her husband." Children are wanted as a source of support, comfort in old age and power against enemies.

Practically none of the responding mothers who showed the desire to have more children defined how many more children they wanted. An unpublished ARAMCO survey in the Eastern Province showed that six children is the desired number among villagers; male children were preferred. Dickson[8] said in 1959; "Every Arabian woman's greatest desire in life is to have a child. She will be divorced if she does not produce a son and heir for her husband."

There is no statistically significant difference in the response of the mothers to the question "How many more children do you want to have?" according to their age group, number of previous marriages or number of previous pregnancies.

Mothers were asked if a woman could prevent pregnancy (Table 1).

Table 1. Percentage Distribution of Mothers Responding to the Question "Can A Woman Prevent Pregnancy?"

Community	No. of Respondents	Yes (%)	No (%)	Don't know (%)	Total (%)
Settled (A)	79	32	14	54	100
Semi-settled (B)	94	3	10	87	100
Nomadic (C)	73	0	7	93	100
All respondents	246	10	12	78	100

The figures in Table 1 are highly significant. They show clearly that mothers from the settled community are more knowledgeable about the possibility of preventing pregnancy. Approximately 32 percent of them said, "a woman can prevent pregnancy," against 3 percent from the semi-settled and none from the nomadic communities. However, women from the settled community might be more expressive. All those who said contraception is possible mentioned pills as the method, except two women from the settled community who mentioned injections. Although pills are sold freely in Taif, I presume that many of those who mentioned them have never seen them. We interviewed selected knowledgeable people (key informants) in Turaba about family planning and particularly about practiced methods of birth control. Men were always glad to discuss sex and married life in general but when the subject came down to specific questions on birth control, they lost interest. In general, they do not accept contraception, as it is against their beliefs. They always want more children, since children are a sign of wealth, strength and vitality. They reason that it does not cost much, if anything, to have one more child, as he or she will be raised with the other children in the household. In very few cases we found that coitus interruptus was practiced. This was especially the case when the marriage was not successful and on its way to breaking down.

The average number of pregnancies per mother in the three communities is 5.2, with no statistically significant difference between the communities. This is, however, a selected population of mothers who have children under five years and have not completed their families.

A survey conducted in Jordan in 1971 (Rizk, unpublished) showed the average number of children to be 5.6 for all mothers in that nation. The average number of children ever to be born to a woman during her entire reproductive period, according to the same survey, was between nine and 10; this same figure was found in Palestine in 1945.[9]

In such a community, the question of the possible effects of polygamy upon the family is always raised. Some studies have shown that polygamy does have a negative effect on the fertility of the population.

Family Nutrition

"People like what they eat, rather than eat what they like." Lewin.[10]

The female interviewers questioned the mothers in Turaba about the nutrition of the family as a whole and of the children in particular. Informal open-ended questions were asked to learn more about the cultural values of foods and the customs related to them.

Some difficulties were faced in this part of the study. For instance, in estimating the quantity of rice eaten "yesterday", the mother would demonstrate the quantity either by her hand or by a local home utensil. The interviewer would convert the demonstrated amount into a standardized local measurement "Robaa" (800 gm.) and then to metric measurement. In estimating the quantities consumed per month, we depended on the memory of the respondent. A nutritional survey based on a day-by-day estimation was beyond our ability. The problems of recall, human error of the interviewers, the motivation of the respondents, as well as other problems of reliability and validity of assessment have been faced in many nutritional studies.[11,12]

We asked the mothers about the family consumption of certain types of food "yesterday". The average number of household members participating in the last evening meal was 3.1 adults and 3.4 children, with no difference between the communities. No attempt was made, however, to adjust for the age of children which may go up to 15.

Table 2 shows the percentage of families who mentioned eating specific types of food "yesterday".

Table 2. Percent of Households Who Mentioned Eating Specific Types of Food "Yesterday".

Comm.	Resp.	Meat.	Vegts.	Fruit	Milk	Date	Tea	Coffee
A	77	68	53	16	36	62	51	98
B	117	6	4	--	18	82	78	93
C	80	8	1	--	16	86	78	86

Apparently, families in Souq consumed more meat, vegetables, fruit and milk than families in the other two communities.

This table is probably a good reflection of the difference of the nutritional status of the three communities.

People in Souq consume more varieties of foods including meat, vegetables and fruits, while the semi-settled and nomadic communities depend largely on flour, rice, dates and tomato paste with little and occasional variations.

Child Nutrition

Of our respondents, 65 percent in Souq, 94 percent in the semi-settled and 92 percent of the nomads said that they gave their children samna (ghee) at birth for the first three days of life. "It lubricates the intestines, cleans it and gives the child nourishment." If samna is not available, drops of castor oil are given to the baby. A lactating neighbor or relative may be called to breastfeed the baby until the mother lactates in the second or third day. The wet nurse is considered by religious beliefs as the child's second mother and there would be no intermarriage between the two women's children.

Table 3 shows the type of milk fed to the children in the three communities by age group.

Table 3. Type of Milk Feeding of Children in the Study by Age Group.

Comm.	Age Group (Months)	No.	Breast Milk	Powdered Milk	Goat Milk	Weaned
	0-12	33	17	11	2	3
A	13-24	26	12	8	1	5
	24+	104	--	2	1	101
	All ages	163	32	18	4	109
	0-12	39	35	1	1	2
B	13-24	37	26	6	1	4
	24+	118	3	--	--	115
	All ages	194	62	7	2	121
	0-12	29	27	1	--	1
C	13-24	29	22	1	1	5
	24+	102	--	2	--	100
	All ages	160	49	4	1	106

Breast-feeding is the predominant method of feeding children up to two years of age in the three communities. Feeding with powdered milk is one of the main differences in the nutrition of children between the three communities. While 19 (32 percent) of the children less than two years old in Souq are given powdered milk, only seven (9 percent) and two (4 percent) of the same group in the semi-settled and nomadic communities, respectively, are given powdered milk. In Souq, powdered milk is considered a sign of modernization.

In the semi-settled and nomadic communities powdered milk is used occasionally if the mother is sick or the child is unable to suck her breast. A wet nurse, either hired or volunteered, is far more preferable to powdered milk. This is not only because powdered milk is expensive but also because human milk is highly preferable to any other kind of milk. An old Arab proverb says, "Character impressed by the mother's milk cannot be altered by anything except death."

Goat's milk, if available, is given to grown children but rarely to young children, since it is believed to cause "Tukhma" (anorexia and diarrhea). Breast feeding is practiced in the easy-going, self-demand method, a method which is also recommended by some modern authorities. The duty of the mother is to quiet the child with her breast milk and never let him/her cry for a prolonged period of time; otherwise he will get "Bakwa" (an epileptic fit).

Among the people we asked, we did not find discrimination against female babies in breast-feeding. Discrimination does exist, however, in solid food feeding. One of the female interviewers reported that some Bedouin mothers gave their male children the breast for more than 24 months, a longer period than for females. This preference for males over females has been found by Puyet[13] among Arab refugees in Lebanon.

Solid Food

Table 4 shows the age at which semi-solids and solid foods are introduced to children.

Table 4. Percent Distribution of Age of Introducing Solid Foods to Babies.

		Age in Months				
Community	No.	<6	6 -9	10 - 12	>12	Total
A	97	10	54	29	7	100
B	121	23	42	31	4	100
C	101	17	44	33	6	100

Mostly, the introduction of solid food commences at the age of six to nine months. At that age the child is given Al Easha (a piece of bread, rice or a date) to suck on. Gradually the child is given what is available on the food table and at any time of the day. Meat is not given at this time as it is "too heavy" for very young children. A child is allowed to suck meat when he is around one and a half years old, but is not allowed to eat it before the age of two years.

Weaning

The vast majority of mothers (more than 90 percent) in all communities wean their children at exactly two years of age or earlier if they become pregnant again. Weaning here means the cessation of breast-feeding. The milk of a pregnant mother is thought to be toxic to her child. It is believed to cause "Ghoosh" (diarrhea and bulging abdomen). In Souq it appears that weaning before two years (for reasons other than pregnancy) is practiced more than in the other two communities. It is strongly believed that a child must be weaned in the same week or even on the day of becoming two years of age. People believe that this is ordered by God. It has been recommended by the Quran and by the Prophet Mohammed that a child better be weaned at this age, but is never mandatory.[14] Jaliffe[15] mentioned the same belief among people in Lebanon, Syria, Iraq and Morocco. Buck, in his study in Chad, found that 92 percent of the mothers in Djimtito, a predominantly Muslim community, wean their children at two years of age.

Preschool Chidren

After weaning, the two-year-old child is allowed to eat every kind of food available, including meat. At the age of three years the child sits regularly at three meals with the members of the family except the father, who in nomadic and semi-nomadic communities usually eats the noon and evening meals with his neighbors, friends or guests.

At the age of five to seven years, the male child is allowed to join his father except in the presence of strangers. A male child is always highly favored with the best food. "A male child is a much valued arrival in the family, to him is passed the honor of the family, and upon him rests the responsibility of maintaining it," Lipsky[16]

History of Morbidity

Mothers were questioned by the female interviewers concerning the health conditions of their children. They were asked about the presence of four selected complaints; diarrhea, cough, fever and eye disease.

Table 5 shows the prevalence of the four selected complaints among children in the three communities by age group.

Essentially there is no difference in distribution of age groups in the three communities. There is a consistently lower rate of complaints in Souq than in semi-settled and nomadic communities. The difference between semi-settled and nomadic communities is not consistent.

Table 5. Percent Distribution of Children Up to Five Years With Four Selected Complaints.

Age in Months	Community	Number of Children	Diarrhea	Cough	Fever	Eye Disease
	A	33	9	18	9	12
0-11	B	39	8	49	18	28
	C	29	17	34	21	45
	A	26	12	8	15	8
12 - 23	B	37	32	35	22	16
	C	29	24	45	24	34
	A	104	8	14	10	8
24 - 59	B	118	11	41	19	23
	C	102	14	38	12	29
	A	163	9	13	10	9
All Ages	B	194	14	41	19	23
	C	160	16	39	16	33

Table 6 shows the two-week period prevalence of the same four complaints among children. Souq has lower prevalence than the other two communities in all conditions except diarrhea.

Table 6. Percent Distribution of Children Up to Five Years With Two Week History of Four Selected Complaints.

Community	No. of Children	Diarrhea	Cough	Fever	Eye Disease
A	163	22	17	17	12
B	194	24	41	28	31
C	160	19	40	26	29

In summary we can say that there was no difference between the children in the three communities in the incidence of diarrhea. Cough and eye diseases were significantly higher in nomadic and semi-settled communities. Fever was also higher in the latter two communities, but was only of borderline significance.

Infant Mortality Rate (IMR)

Table 7 shows the preceding years live births, number of deaths among children up to one year, and the calculated infant mortality rate.

The apparent difference between the three communities in IMR was not statistically significant at the 5 percent level as the sample size was not large enough to detect such a difference.

Some years ago, Dickson[17] observed that among 15 Bedouin children perhaps only three or four survive.

My personal impression is that these figures are not sufficiently reliable, since our cross sectional study depended a great deal on the memory of the mother. Any future studies on IMR should be based on longitudinal surveys and birth and death registers.

Table 7. Live Births, Infant Deaths And Infant Mortality Rate in the Preceding Year.

Community	No. of Mothers	Live Births	Infant Deaths	IMR/1,000
A	100	47	4	85
B	124	48	8	166
C	108	39	7	179
Total	332	134	19	134

Clinical Examination

Selected clinical signs were chosen as indicators for nutritional and infectious diseases. Table 8 shows the prevalence of these selected conditions among the children up to five years old. There is no apparent difference in the prevalence of the conditions between the three communities except in ulcers (p = < 0.01) and infected penis (p = <0.005), also noted no obvious difference between males and females in any of the three communities except in pediculosis and conjunctivitis which were always higher among females.

Malnutrition: The prevalence of the clinical signs of malnutrition, such as hair depigmentation, nasolabial seborrhea and angular stomatitis is not significantly different in the three communities (p = < 0.030).

There was a total of 21 children with one or more positive clinical signs of malnutrition (hair depigmentation, nasolabial seborrhea, angular stomatitis and leg edema). Out of these, five were cases who had more than one important clinical sign of kwashiorkor. There were no indications of any linkage of malnutrition with the sex of the child.

Due to the small number of observed conditions, no definite correlation between the prevalence of the condition and the age of the children could be determined except in a few cases. In all communities, no sign of nutritional deficiency was observed in children under one year of age. The same is true of pediculosis. Conjunctivitis has a relatively high prevalence among children below one year of age - 33 percent of all cases in Souq, 49 percent in semi-settled and 42 percent in nomadic community. Smallpox scars were found on 35 children in Souq, 21 children in semi-settled, and nine chilren in the nomadic community.

Table 8. Percent Distribution of Positive Clinical Findings Among Children Up to Five Years.

Community	A	B	C
Respondents	101	133	98
Clinical Findings			
Hair depigmentation	2	2	4
Nasolabial seborrhea	2	1	1
Angular stomatitis	3	2	3
Acute conjunctivitis	12	14	19
Ulcers	2	11	8
Infected penis	––	8	7
Pediculosis	21	15	21
Liver enlargement	4	4	3
Spleen enlargement	––	––	––
Leg edema	2	8	5
Marasmus	2	4	3

The lack of differences between the three communities in the prevalence of the clinical signs of malnutrition does not reflect the anthropometric findings which will be discussed later, for it shows a significant difference between Souq and the nomadic community.

Other nutritional studies indicate that the clinical findings, being insensitive, do not always reflect the nutritional status of a population.[18,19] Although some typical cases of kwashiorkor have been seen in this study, sub-clinical cases might exist undiagnosed.[20] Infantile beri beri, an expected condition in communities B and C which depend largely on polished rice as the main staple food, might have already led to some infantile deaths.

Conjunctivitis is less prevalent in this dry part of the country than in the Eastern Province where trachoma affects 90 percent of the school-age and older children.[21] Conjunctival scarring as entropion and ectropion was not revealed. However, the absence of gross scarification does not exclude the possibility of the existence of trachoma in a community.[22]

Ulcers and Infected Penis: Ulcers observed are either traumatic or the result of infected cautery. Infected penis in all observed cases was the result of an unhygienic process of circumcising young male children. Although cautery and circumcision are practiced at homes in all communities, the observed favorable outcome of both procedures in Souq might be due to more sterile techniques, better post-operative hygiene or the availability of antibacterial drugs in the Health Center.

Anthropometric Measurements

The manner in which height, weight, head circumference and chest circumference change with age in months was determined according to the least squares polynomial equation.

There is a significant difference between the children in the three communities in weight and height. The differences are largely between females in the settled and nomadic communities. This difference might be due to the preference for males over females in the nomadic community. The difference between male and female measurements was also found by Morley in West Africa.[23]

The weights of children, males and females, in the settled and nomadic communities are plotted together with the Harvard Standard[24] (50 percentile) as a standard of reference (Figure 9).

A similar deviation from the Boston Standard was observed by Taha[25] among Sudanese children, sexes combined.

Normally, the chest to head ratio exceeds one after six months of age.[26] In our population this predicted ratio exceeds one among males only at the age of three years, whereas among females it remains below one even at that age. This might indicate a low nutritional status and hindrance to normal growth, especially among females.

Laboratory Investigations

Hemoglobin:

Table 9 shows the percentage distribution of the hemoglobin value in gm. percent among the studied group of children up to five years in the three communities. The children in Souq have a higher percentage of readings above 10 gm. percent. If a hemoglobin level of less than 10 gm. percent is taken as an indication of anemia,[27] this would indicate a higher prevalence of anemia among young children in semi-settled and nomadic communities.

X^2 test has been applied to differences in the Hg value less than 10 gm. percent between communities A and C. The difference is significant ($p = < 005$).

Table 9. Percent Distribution of Children Up to Five Years by Level of Hemoglobin in gms.

Comm.	No. of Children	Hemoglobin gm%						Cumulative Readings		Total
		4+	6+	8+	10+	12+	14+	-- 10	10+	
A	95		3	15	41	36	5	18	82	100
B	123	1	12	22	43	21	1	35	65	100
C	90		10	24	50	12	3	34	66	100

* Reading in 10ths but chartered to nearest whole figure.

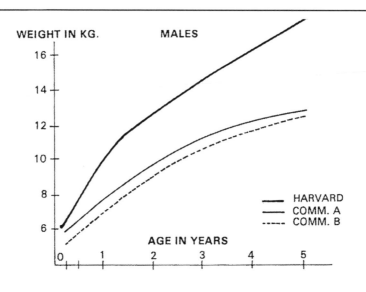

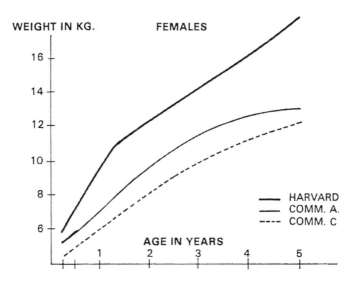

Figure 9. **PREDICTED WEIGHT FOR MALES AND FEMALES 0-5 YEARS IN TURABA COMPARED TO HARVARD STANDARD (50th PERCENTILE)**

Malaria:

Malaria thin and thick smears from 135 school children were negative on microscopic examination. In discussion with the key informants in Turaba, many mentioned "Homma Al Thuluth" (the fever which comes every third day) with chilling and ends with enlarged spleen. The fever was prevalent in Turaba 12 years ago at the time of "Al Haia" - the rain. It was the great killer of children at that time.

Treponema Palledum Test: (See Health Problems pp. 131-139)

Cholera Vibriocedal Antibodies: 98 samples of sera were examined for cholera vibriocedal antibodies. Of 41 samples of sera examined from Souq, 27 (65 percent) showed positive results for Ogawa strain, Enaba strain, or both. Among 57 samples of sera examined from communities B and C, 32 (56 percent) were positive. In Souq, 15 sera (55 percent of total positive sera) had a titer of more than 620, while in communities B and C, 12 sera (36 percent of total positive sera) showed the same titer.

Historically no cholera has been reported in Makkah (the possible point of entry of cholera to Hejaz area in West Saudi Arabia) since 1912.[28] This would tend to exclude the existence of clinical or even sub-clinical cases which might be found in endemic areas. The possibilities for the prevalence of cholera antibodies among the examined population are previous vaccination of infection with non-specific antigen.

Intestinal Parasites:

Table 10 shows the results of stool examination of children from Souq and communities B and C combined.

Table 10. Percent Distribution of Children Up to Five Years with Intestinal Parasites (Communities B & C Combined).

Comm.	Number	With Infection	E. coli	H. nana	G. lamblia
A	87	40	19	15	14
B, C	99	43	20	16	26

Two pathogenic organisms, H.nana and G.lamblia, beside E.coli were found. Approximately half of the children in both communities were infected by one or more of the organisms. Seven children in Souq and 17 children in B and C had multiple infection. All children less than one year old were negative.

No apparent aggregation of cases in individual households was observed. Children in 42 houses in all communities (with two or more chilren per house) were examined for intestinal parasites. In 11 of these households (26 percent) more than one child was positive, in 20 households (48 percent) one child was positive and the other was negative, and in 11 households (26 percent) both were negative.

E. coli is almost equally prevalent in both communities. Although it is a non-pathogenic organism, its presence is concrete evidence that the host has injected fecal material.

Two school children living in Alawa complained of blood in the stool, and on stool examination Schistosoma mansoni eggs were revealed. Alawa village, five miles from Souq, is a known epidemic focus for schistosoma mansoni. In the summer of 1965, in a screening survey for schistosomiasis in Turaba, 32 stools were collected from Alawa children. Fourteen were positive on direct smear and an additional four on sedimentation of the entire stool.[29]

The results of the stool examination in our study were felt to be on the low side. The collected samples were preserved in MIF stain (Merthiolate-Iodine Formalin) for three months before they were examined. This could have affected the results.

Rectal Swabs:

Forty-four rectal swabs were examined bacteriologically. None of the material was positive for Shigella and Salmonella organisms. The absence of Shigella and Salmonella does not seem to be contradictory to the prevalence of diarrhea among the children under the study. Many cases of acute diarrhea usually lack a definable infectious agent.

Tuberculin Tine Test:

Figure 10 shows the results of the Tine Test, by age group and sex in 269 persons in community A and 118 persons in communities B and C combined. Communities B and C show a higher prevalence of positive reactions (2mm and more) than community A among age group under 19 years, and more or less a similar prevalence among those over 20 years. Females in both communities have a higher prevalence than males in age group under 19 years and less prevalence among those over 22 years.

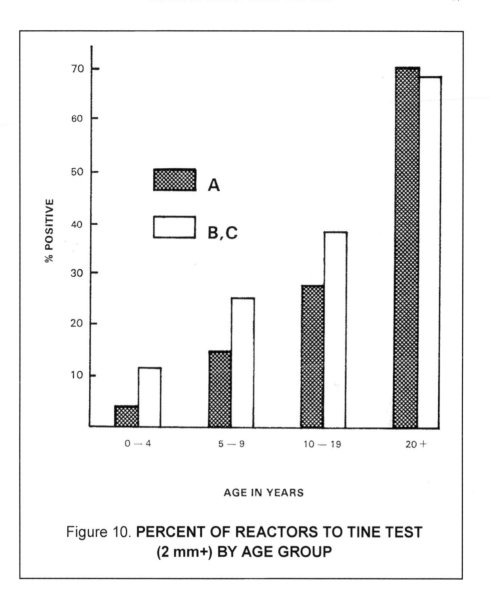

Figure 10. **PERCENT OF REACTORS TO TINE TEST (2 mm+) BY AGE GROUP**

TURABA IN 1981

Changing Turaba

In 1981, a visit was made to observe the changes in Turaba and to asses the health services system and where it stands in contributing to the promotion of the health of the people.

No reliable demographic data is available for Turaba as expected in a community with continuous mobility, settlement and migration to and from cities. The estimated population of Turaba is 45,000 people (compared with 30,000 in 1967), 20 percent of whom are still nomadic Bedouins.

Almost every aspect of life has changed in Turaba since the last visit. Souq, the main village, is unrecognizable for it has become a small modern town. The mud houses have been replaced by concrete buildings and have increased tenfold in number. The dirt roads have become asphalt streets and the half dozen small shops have been replaced by several modern markets. Electricity, telephones and color television sets are now a feature in almost every house.

Changes abound in the small settlement areas (Hejar) around Souq. They have increased in number and size, most are now accessible by asphalt roads and most of the mud houses and huts have been demolished and replaced by modern concrete buildings.

The most amazing changes have taken place in the desert. A Bedouin family, although still living in a tent, uses butane gas for cooking and may own a small pickup truck, usually driven by the housewife or her daughter. The Bedouin woman is probably the only female driver in Saudi Arabia. A Bedouin herdsman feeds his herd with inexpensive barley which is subsidized by the government. He also brings water in tanks to his location, and his livestock is taken to the market in a Mercedes truck. As a result he does not need to roam around as much as before looking for grass and water.

In general the average income of the family in Turaba has increased several fold over the last 15 years. The family may have more than one source of income including farming, trade, government employment, animal husbandry (goats, sheep and camels), social security and financial support from young adults working in the cities.

The sudden economic improvement in Turaba, as in most parts of the country, started in the mid-1970s triggered by the tremendous increase in oil prices. In 1976, the government also initiated a system of giving free loans of up to SR300,000 to landowners in Turaba for the building of houses. In five years, more than 2,500 concrete houses were built and 1,500 more are planned within the next two years. Other factors contributing to the process of economic development were the establishment of a 140 kilometer asphalt road to Taif, the introduction of electricity and telephones to Souq and, in the last two years, an increase in the rate of rainfall after a long period of drought.

The economic improvement has been accompanied by social changes. In the late 1960s there were four schools for boys and one for girls. Now there are 17 boys schools and three girls schools and more are planned. Adult education for both men and women is in the process of development.

The social change shows itself in Ergain, a small settlement area (Hejrat) established in the late 1960s. The 100 or so mud houses and huts have given way to more than 300 block and concrete buildings.

The people of Ergain, with the guidance of their wise old Sheikh, Menahi Al Gharmool, have built two small one-story buildings - one a school with a teacher provided by the Department of Education, and the other a dispensary for which they are requesting a physician from the Department of Health. A co-operative committee was established and currently runs a bakery, grocery, petrol pump and a small generator which supplies electricity six hours a day to 30 percent of the houses. The people themselves helped in paving parts of the 20 kilometer rough and rocky road to Souq.

Eating habits have changed. Rice and bread still constitute their staple diet, but an average family can now purchase lamb or beef (which for them is the most precious food because "it maintains health and gives power and vitality") or chicken almost every day. Milk, butter and dates are produced locally in sufficient quantities. Eggs and vegetables are available but seldom consumed as their nutritional values are not recognized. In the local grocery, more than one brand of powdered milk is available for baby feeding, for to the villagers this is a sign of modernization, a phenomenon observed in other developing societies.[30,31]

The people of Ergain are becoming more oriented towards "modern medicine" but health services are still not easily accessible (more than 80 percent of the attendants at Souq Health Center come from a radius of ten kilometers). As in the case of the rest of Turaba, they still seek folk medicine for many of their ailments.

Fifteen years ago their main demands from the government were simple - a dispensary staffed by a nurse, a boys school and a mosque. Their demands at present include an asphalt road to Souq, a bridge over the wadi (the water bed separating Ergain from the main road to Turaba), a doctor to staff the health center, public electricity and a girls school. According to their Sheikh, "out of ignorance and prejudice we resisted for years the opening of a girls school in our Hejrat, but now we ask for it because we see its relevance in the life of our women."

The socioeconomic development in Turaba has most likely led to an improvement in the health of the people in general and the young children in particular through improved nutrition, housing and education. It has its adverse aspects, such as the increase in the number of road accidents, artificial feeding for babies and the increased pressure of life.

The main question that remains to be answered is, "How has the health center contributed to the improvement of the health of the people in the last 15 years?"

The Health Center

The health center in Turaba is still part of the Development Center (DC) which is composed of four units: Education, Social Welfare, Health and Agriculture. The DC is sponsored and supervised by the Ministry of Social Welfare.

In 1967, the health center in Souq was staffed by one Pakistani physician and four health assistants - a pharmacy assistant, a female nurse/midwife, a male nurse and a heath inspector (the only Saudi member). The health center was the only provider of primary health services for the 30,000 inhabitants, and the secondary point of contact was Taif, 140 kilometers away by paved, but not asphalted road. The center was attended by an average of 95 outpatients per day, most coming from within a radius of five kilometers. The services offered were exclusively curative.

In 1981, the health center in Souq was staffed by three physicians, a dentist and 10 health assistants. The center is the main provider of primary health care for 45,000 people and is attended by an average of 325 outpatients per day.

The functions of the health center in Souq will be described under two headings - curative and preventive aspects.

A. Curative Aspects

During one week, 1,787 patients attended the health center, a daily average of 325 (an average of 108 patients per day per physician). In addition, 17 patients are seen daily by the dentist. Fifteen percent of the patients are expatriate (Egyptians, Pakistanis, Indians and Yemenis), and most are unskilled laborers.

Table 11 shows the distribution by age and sex of the 1,787 outpatients attending the health center during one week. The proportion of males to females is almost equal. The under five-year-old age group constitutes 16.8 percent of the total, which is a rather low figure in a community where the under-five age group makes up approximately 20 percent of the population and is considered an at-risk group.

A patient coming to the health center may select his/her doctor as there is no registration, record system or screening. Eighty percent of the females go to the female doctor, whereas all male patients (over five years) go to the male doctors.

The two male physicians were observed for three hours in their clinics. The average time spent by each one of them seeing a patient was one minute and one second. The doctor would listen to the patient's complaint, put his hand on the wrist of the patient and occasionally touch his chest with the stethoscope. At the same time, he enters the patient's name, age and diagnosis in his log book, writes the prescription and hands it over to the patient. The writing takes a good part of his time.

No patient was adequately examined since there was no couch, sphygmomanometer or thermometer in the examining room.

Table 11. Distribution of 1,787 Outpatients Who Attended the Health Center Over a One-Week Period, by Age and Sex.

| | Age Group in Years | | | |
	<5years	5 to 15 years	>1 5 years	Total
Male	148	97	677	922
Female	152	96	617	865
Total	300	193	1,294	1,787

The diagnosis, or rather the impression of the physician, follows a symptomatic pattern. Table 12 shows the distribution of diagnosis of 1,787 cases seen by the three physicians over a one-week period. The differences observed between men and women in cardiovascular, eye and skin diseases are more likely to be differences in judgement.

Table 12. Distribution of Diagnosis of 1,787 Cases Recorded Collectively by Three Physicians During One Week.

Diagnosis	Children (<5 years)	Men	Women	Total	%
Gasterintestinal diseases	55	65	122	242	13.5
Chest diseases	78	110	83	271	15.2
Cardiovascular diseases	--	5	23	28	1.6
Nervous system diseases	--	14	31	45	2.5
Eye diseases	21	65	25	111	6.2

E.N.T. diseases	50	50	60	160	9.0
Bone & muscle diseases	2	158	196	356	19.9
Skin diseases	38	85	28	151	8.4
Genito-urinary diseases	––	39	48	87	4.9
Infectious diseases	10	6	6	22	1.2
Common cold	15	98	41	154	8.6
Others	31	79	50	160	9.6
Total	300	774	713	1,787	100.0

Table 13 shows the drugs prescribed for these 1,787 patients over a one-week period. The average number of drugs prescribed for a patient is three. Multivitamins, analgesics and antibiotics are freely dispensed, together they constitute 74 percent of all drugs dispensed (indiscriminate polypharmacy). Non-specific drugs such as hormones (mainly testosterone for old men seeking sexual vitality) and cortisone derivitives have a higher ratio compared to more specific drugs such as antidiabetics and hypotensives. Antibiotics (including penbritin, tetracycline and streptomycin) are dispensed frequently in rather small doses. A patient may be given one injection of antibiotics and a two-day supply of eight capsules.

Table 13. Distribution of Drugs Prescribed for 1,787 Outpatients in One Week.

Items	Tablets	Injections	Other Forms	Total	%
Analgesics	1,054	––	147	1,201	21.8
Vitamins	831	515	89	1,453	26.0
Antibiotics & Sulpha	640	223	575	1,438	26.1
Cortisone derivatives	128	14		142	2.6
Hormones	43	17		60	1.1
Antimalaria	19	32		51	0.9
Antidiabetics	3			3	0.05
Hypotensives	3			3	0.05
Others	589	165	428	1,128	21.4
Total	3,310	966	1,239	5,515	100.0

Injections are highly favored by most of the patients - "it goes directly to the blood." Colored injections and calcium bromate (for the warm sensation it gives) are also in high demand. The physician prescribes medicine in injection form (even as one ampule of streptomycin) to satisfy the patient, or as one of the physicians put it "a psychological treatment for the patient." A Bedouin attendant can even get a Vitamin B complex injection prescribed for his sister who does not feel well at home.

Three prescription sheets selected at random from the pharmacy clearly show the indiscriminate dispensing of drugs.

1. Diagnosis: Conjuctivitis.

    Streptomycin - one amp.
    Aspirin - six tablets.
    Eye ointment - one tube.

2. Diagnosis: Headache.

    Aspirin - six tablets.
    Multivitamin - six tablets.
    Buscopan - one injection.

3. Chronic Bronchitis.

    Streptomycin - two amp.
    Aspirin - eight tablets.
    Multivitamin - eight tablets.
    Aminophylline - eight tablets.
    Penbritin - 250 mg., eight caps.

The clinical work is backed by laboratory and radiological services which, although available, are not utilized effectively.

Out of 325 patients attending the health center each day the laboratory technician performed an average of eight simple routine examinations: three urine, three stool and two blood.

The dentist treats an average 17 patients per day. Out of 94 patients seen over one week, 66 percent had teeth extractions.

According to the dentist, the population of Turaba has a high rate of dental morbidity. A man or woman at the age of 25 years has a third of his/her teeth either missing or with caries. This is most probably because of the high consumption of dates and lack of oral hygiene.

The health center also takes care of emergency cases such as simple wounds, burns or scorpion stings. The health center refers approximately 15 cases every month to Taif Hospital. However, no follow-up of the cases or feedback from the hospital is ensured.

An inspector would come from the Department of the Regional Health Services in Taif for a one or two day visit, two or three times a year for general inspection and to solve emerging administrative problems.

B. Preventive Aspects

The estimated birth rate in Turaba is 45 per thousand, i.e. 2,025 live births per year for a population of 45,000. By law, a child should receive full immunization against poliomylitis, DPT and tuberculosis before a birth certificate is issued. Because a birth certificate is not usually needed until school entry at the age of six years, a busy or dilatory father can delay its issue for years provided he pays a penalty of 10 Riyals.

For the expected 2,025 newly born children in 1980, 640 birth certificates were issued from the health center in Souq, the only place from which birth certificates are issued in Turaba. Only 258 children had received complete doses of poliomylitis and triple vaccines during the same year. This is 40 percent of the 640 registered newborn and only 12.7 percent of the 2,025 expected newborn.

There is no record of the age at which a child receives the first or subsequent immunization since there are no individual cards for the vaccines. BCG was given to 772 children during the first week of life. No other vaccines are being given, except when a mass vaccination against meningitis was carried out in 1980.

In the health center's refrigerator we found an ample quantity of BCG and diptheria vaccines which had already expired, as well as measles vaccines which would expire within the month.

Last year, 208 pregnant women (average 17 per month) visited the health center for general complaints. Each had been seen by the female doctor, who examined her blood pressure and ordered a urine test for sugar and albumen. No follow-up programs were carried out.

The midwife is called eventually to attend the delivery of a woman at her home (a delivering mother is usually assisted by an older, experienced woman relative or neighbor). Last year the nurse/midwife attended 279 deliveries at homes out of 2,025 expected deliveries (14 percent). There were no deliveries at the health center. Although a few mothers would be expected to go to the hospital at Taif, there are no records available to verify this.

No other forms of maternal and child health acvities such as health education, nutrition, early detection of cases, neonatal or postnatal care take place.

The doctors in the health center are, by law, not permitted to make home visits, although some hidden private practice does occur.

School health for boys is the responsibility of the school health department under the Ministry of Education. One single physician works in Turaba and is responsible for 17 boys schools with more than 2,000 pupils. The physician pays one or two visits a year to each school. In that one-day visit he makes a general inspection and treats the sick.

Environmental sanitation is the responsibility of the municipality. Even the cleanliness of the health center building and its surroundings does not come under the jurisdiction of the doctors in the health center or their assistants. The main responsibilities of the two sanitarian assistants are to record the outpatient statistics and complete official forms for the Ministry of Health. They eventually vaccinate children when accompanied by their fathers. Last year they participated in a program for installing 160 latrines in the villages.

Schistosomiasis is a recognized problem in Turaba but its epidemiology has not yet been studied. In a survey carried out last year among an unidentified number of school children in Souq, 32 students were found positive for Schistosoma mansoni. A schistosomiasis control team from Taif visits Turaba every four to six months for general survey and treatment. At the time of our visit, the team was completing a 12-day survey (planned and operated by the team from Taif) which covered 700 individuals. The survey recorded 15 positive cass, all natives, with Schistosoma mansoni and one Egyptian laborer with Schistosoma hematobium. Patients were treated by the schistosomiasis team with no reference made to the health center. Of 97 wells previously reported positive for Biomphlaria species, treated with molluscides (Moltox) and re-examined at this time, 28 were positive indicating inefficient control measures.

The example of Turaba presents a lesson worth learning when planning for the future. The study indicates that the expansion of health services by increasing the number of health units and personnel does not necessarily bring about an improvement in health.

The expansion of health services should be accompanied by a better understanding of the life style of the people, health ecology and appropriate utilization of health resources, especially human.

In Chapter V (page 181) we will discuss a plan of action to improve the primary health care in Turaba.

BIBLIOGRAPHY

1. Sebai ZA. The Health of the Family in a Changing Arabia. 3rd Ed. Jeddah: Tihama Publications, 1983.

2. Sebai ZA, Miller D, Ba'ageel H. Study of Three Health Centers in Rural Saudi Arabia. Saudi Medical Journal 1980: 1;4.

3. Miller DL, Sebai ZA. Health Center in Khulais. In: Proceedings of the 5th Saudi Annual Medical Meeting, Riyadh University, Faculty of Medicine, 1980.

4. Banoub S. Primary Health Care in Qasim. In: Sebai ZA. Ed. Community Health In Saudi Arabia. A Profile of Two Villages in the Qasim Region.

Saudi Medical Journal Monograph No. 1. Great Britain: Stanhope Press, 1982: 59-70.

5. Sebai ZA. Ed. Community Health in Saudi Arabia: A Profile of Two Villages in the Qasim Region. Saudi Medical Journal Monograph No. 1. Great Britain: Stanhope Press, 1982: 71-76.

6. Sebai ZA. Health Manpower Development in Yemen Arab Republic. WHO Assignment Report 1976; EM/HMD/359.

7. Sebai ZA. Health Manpower Development in Oman. WHO Assignment Report 1978; EM/HMD/394.

8. Dickson HRP. The Arab of the Desert; A Glimpse into Bedoiun Life in Kuwait and Saudi Arabia. London: Allen and Unwin, 1959: 190.

9. Patai R. Golden River to Golden Road; Society, Culture and Change in the Middle East. Philadelphia: University of Pennsylvania Press, 1962: 84.

10. Lewin K. Factors Behind Food Habits and Methods of Change. Bulletin National Research Council 1943; 108.

11. Taha SA. Ecological Factors Underlying Protein-Calorie Malnutrition in an Irrigated Area of the Sudan. Ecology of Food and Nutrition 1979; 7:193-201.

12. Gersovitz M, Madden JP, Smiciklas-Wright H. Validity of the 24 Hour Dietry Recall and Seven Day Record for Group Comparisons. Journal of American Dietetic Association July 1978: 73.

13. Puyet JH. et al. Nutritional and Growth Characteristics of Arab Refugee Children in Lebanon. American Journal of Clinical Nutritional 1963; 13: 145-157.

14. Quran II: 233.

15. Jelliffe DB. Infant Nutrition in the Subtropics and Tropics. 2nd Ed. Geneva: WHO, 1968: 27-37 (WHO Monograph Ser. No. 29).

16. Lipsky GA. Saudi Arabia; Its People, Its Solity, Its Culture. New Haven: H.R.A.F. Press 1959: 297.

17. Dickson HRP. ibid.

18. James WPT. Kwashiorkor and Marasmus: Old Concepts and New Developments. In: Proceedings Royal Society of Medicine Sept. 1977; 70.

19. Jelliffe DB. Assessment of Nutritional Status of the Community. Geneva: WHO, 1966: (WHO Monograph Ser. No. 53).

20. WHO Expert Committee on Medical Assessment of Nutritional Status. Geneva: WHO, 1963: (WHO Technical Report Series No. 258).

21. Murray ES. et al. Agents Recovered from Acute Conjunctivitis Cases in Saudi Arabia. American Journal Ophthamology 1957; 43 (4 Pt 2): 32.

22. Haddad NA. Trachoma in Lebanon; Observation on Epidemiology in Rural Areas. American Journal of Medicine and Hygiene 1965; 14: 652-655.

23. Morley DC. et al. Heights and Weights of West African Village Children from Birth to Age of Five. West African Medical Journal Feb. 1968.

24. Nelson WE. Textbook of Paediatrics. 8th Ed. Philadelphia: W.B. Saunders, 1965: 49.

25. Taha SA. Prevalence and Severity of Protein-Calorie Malnutrition in Sudanese Children. Tropical Pediatrics and Environmental Child Health: October 1978.

26. Joint FAO/WHO Technical Meeting on Methods of Planning and Evaluation in Applied Nutrition Programs: Report. Geneva: WHO, 1966: (WHO Tech. Rep. Ser. No. 340).

27. Jelliffe DB. ibid.

28. Pollitzer R. Cholera. Geneva: WHO 1959: (WHO Monograph Ser. No. 43) 63.

29. Alio IS. Epidemiology of Schistosomiasis in Saudi Arabia with Emphasis on Geographical Distribution Pattern. ARAMCO, Dhahran 1967.

30. Carbello M. Fertility Regulation During Human Lactation. WHO Collaborative Studies on Breast-Feeding. Journal Biosocial Science 1977; Suppl. 4): 83-89.

31. Taha SA. Ecological Factors Underlying Protein-Calorie Malnutrition in an Irrigated Area of the Sudan. Ecology of Food and Nutrition 1979; 7: 193-201.

II - KHULAIS

A field project was carried out in Khulais in 1977. It demonstrates the participation of medical students in community diagnosis and delivery of health services in a rural area. Twenty five fourth-year medical students and seven medical professionals carried out the project as a part of the training program in community medicine. The objectives were a combination of education, research and services.

This chapter discusses the educational aspect of the project and the function of the health center. For details of the findings, the reader can refer to Bayoumi et al,[1] Miller and Sebai,[2] Saha et al,[3] and Sebai, Miller and Ba'Aqeel.[4]

The Educational Aspect

The main objective was for the students to develop certain skills: (1) learning to measure the health status of a community; (2) analyzing and interpreting epidemiological data; (3) delivering selected health services; (4) developing the ability to work as a team. Certain concepts were also to be verified: the participation of various agencies including the community in maintaining a health program, using the health center as a base for community health development and the interrelationship between man's health and his environment.

A steering committee of four students was elected at the beginning of the planning stage to coordinate the various activities of the group. Objectives were defined, a protocol established and a household questionnaire and clinical and anthropometric forms were designed and tested. The students were trained to elicit selected clinical signs, take anthropometric measurements and conduct household interviews.

The project was planned and carried out jointly between the faculty of Medicine, King Saud University and the Ministry of Health to ensure the project conformed with the actual health needs of the community. Several organizations contributed to the project, including the Ministries of Interior, Education and Social Welfare and the Department of Girls Education.

Khulais district (Figure 11) was selected as the site of the project. The district is composed of six clusters of villages. The 18,000 inhabitants has a small minority of Bedouins and Negroes. The district was selected because of its limited population and the existence of a health center to function as a base for the project. It is sufficiently remote to demonstrate the problems of health care in a rural community, yet reasonably accessible for the transport of a large team and equipment.

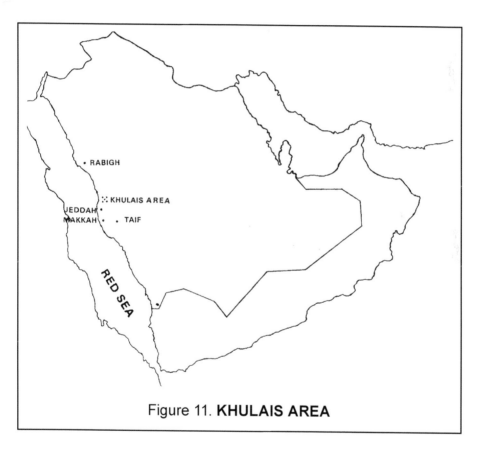

Figure 11. **KHULAIS AREA**

The professional staff consisted of three staff members from King Saud Faculty of Medicine, a phatologist from King Abdul Aziz Faculty of Medicine, a visiting professor from The Middlesex Hospital, London, and two experts in malaria and schistosomiasis from the Ministry of Health. A cinemaphotographer and his assistant, and several health assistants accompanied the team. In Khulais, the local physician and his staff became members of the team. The mobilization of these human resources and the coordination of their work demanded time and effort. Nevertheless, it was an educational experience for students and staff alike.

The day of our arrival at Khulais was Friday. After the mid-day prayer, the project director addressed an audience of several hundred men gathered for prayer from all the villages. He explained the purpose and methods of the project.

Short visits were made to the emir (governor), the headmasters of the schools and several leaders in their homes. Over the traditional Arabic coffee and dates, the project and its implications were discussed. These initial contacts proved to be very helpful in gaining the understanding and cooperation of the people.

The Project Activities

The 25 students were divided into four groups. Each group participated, under supervision, in two or more of the following activities.

- Clinical examination, anthropometric measurements and laboratory investigations of a sample of school children.

- Household survey on socioeconomic, nutritional and environmental conditions.

- Epidemiological studies of malaria and schistosomiasis.

- Health education and immunization program.

Clinical Examination and Anthropometric measurements:

The sample size was determined by the capacity of the team to examine a certain number of children. It was estimated that 50 children could be examined clinically and anthropometrically per day. A total of 280 children was then selected randomly from the primary schools in Khulais town and two surrounding villages, Khwar and Ghran. The examinations were done in the health center in Khulais town.

Each child was examined clinically for signs of malnutrition (depigmentation of hair, nasolabial seborrhea, angular stomatitis, xerosis, conjunctivitis and edema of the lower extremities), eye and skin infection, enlargement of the spleen and liver, and cautery scars. The teeth were examined for florosis pigmentation. Personal data and a short history of illnesses were recorded. The child was then measured for height, weight, and head and arm circumferences.

Laboratory Investigations

A number of laboratory tests were performed on each child, including an examination of urine and stool for ova and parasites and blood tests for malaria parasites, hemoglobin estimation, red blood cell sickling and glucose-6-phosphate dehydrogenase deficiency (G6PD). Other tests (blood grouping, hemoglobin electrophoresis, and estimation of total serum proteins) were carried out later at the University Hospital. Hemoglobin was assayed by the cyanmethemoglobin method according to Dacie & Lewis.[5] The metabisulphite slide test was used for sickling. The brilliant cresyl blue (BCB) screening test for G-6-PD deficiency was performed according to Motulsky & Campbell-Kraut.[6]

The clinical, anthropometric and laboratory findings were recorded on a pre-coded and serially numbered sheet for each child. Children who needed medical care were referred to the local doctor.

Household Survey

A household survey was carried out in more than 210 houses. In the absence of a detailed map of Khulais or any means of identifying dwellings, a structured random sample of households could not easily be obtained. Households were, therefore, chosen by selection of clusters of homes in the various parts of three villages.

The questionnaire covered aspects of the socioeconomic status of the family: knowledge, attitude and practice of health; history of morbidity and mortality; and family nutrition. Two male school teachers and three female nurses from the community were trained on location to help interview household heads and mothers.

Epidemiology of Malaria and Schistosomiasis

A group of students went into the field to study the epidemiology of malaria and schistosomiasis. They collected snail vectors and adult mosquitoes and larvee, obtained finger blood from a sample of village children and learned the technique of applying insecticides, larvacides and mulluscocides. Group discussions were conducted en route.

Health Education and Immunization

The health education activity was a thrilling experience. Several 16mm color films on topics ranging from tuberculosis control to water sanitation were projected in schools and common market places to audiences exceeding 100 at a time. Films in English were explained by the students through a loud speaker. In the schools, a short test on the film topic was made before and after its showing, to assess the gain in knowledge. A female teacher was trained to project the films for the girls in school.

A program of vaccination against diptheria, pertussis and tetanus (DPT) and poliomylitis for preschool children was carried out. Two female schoolteachers were trained to help in administering the vaccination. A list of the names of the vaccinated children was given to the local physician for use in administering booster doses.

Other Activities

At the end of each day, students had to tabulate and analyze the collected data. In the evenings, plenary meetings were held to discuss the day's work and problems faced, as well as the next day's program. The students had to organize such daily activities as transportation, water supply, cleaning, and food purchasing.

An evaluation of the health center function took place concurrently. The students had the opportunity to observe a traditional healer and discuss with him his art. A 16mm color documentary film was produced for educational purposes.

Summary and Conclusion

The main object of this epidemiological/clinical project was to give the students an appreciation of the need for team work and to cultivate their interest in community health.

The planning and organization of such a project is a major undertaking. This is particularly because of the various groups involved, the diversity of their backgrounds and because it is virtually impossible to rectify omissions in the field remote from any sophisticated supply base.

The people of Khulais were highly cooperative and enthusiastic. Many members, including the local doctor and his staff, teachers and community leaders, participated in the activities. A sense of awareness has been raised among the participants and the community.

Very few clinical signs of malnutrition were elicited among the school children. However, a high proportion of mild to moderate stunting and wasting compared to the 50th percentile of Boston children was observed. This could be partially due to racial differences. The stool examination of the school children showed a variety of ovae including Taenia saginata, Entamoeba histolytica, Hymenolepis nana and Ascariasis. No schistosoma ovae were found. The blood examination revealed 15 percent rate of glucose-6-phosphatase dehydrogenase deficiency. Ethrocytic sickling was found in 2.8 percent of the studied population. Malaria parasites were not found.

Toward the end of the period, a questionnaire was distributed among the students asking for their evaluation of the project. Their main responses to a question on the benefits gained from the project were (1) a better understanding of the health problems in a rural Saudi community, (2) experience in conducting a health survey, and (3) learning to work as a team. The findings of the project were presented by the students in a two-day seminar. Some students planned to participate in field work programs during their summer vacation.

By taking the medical students out into the field to work through the health center and by reaching out to the people and functioning as a team, they have developed a positive attitude towards their role as health promoters in their future careers.

Evaluation of the Health Center

A full evaluation of the health center activity would include an assessment of the health needs of the community which it serves, an appraisal of the efficiency of the health center and measurements of its effectiveness in improving the health status of the community. A study of this magnitude could not have been achieved within the time and resources available. Our evaluation, therefore, was based upon ad hoc parameters of the services rather than on any outcome assessment.

The health center is located in a 12-room, single-story building in Khulais town. It is poorly ventilated and dark. The fabric is evidently old and in a poor state of repair.

There is a piped water supply and main electricity, but lighting is poor and standards of hygiene are unsatisfactory with only one wash basin (in the passage) and one toilet for the entire health center.

Most of the furnishings and equipment in use are old and depreciated. However, many of the rooms contain quantities of modern furniture and high quality modern equipment, some of it still in its packing.

The staff at the center consists of a doctor assisted by two female nurses (one midwife), a male nurse, a pharmacist, an X-ray technician, a laboratory assistant, an ambulance driver and two servants.

The Activities

The work of the health center is focused primarily on personal health care to residents of Khulais and a wide area around it. The services provided are mainly acute care of outpatients, but also include some domiciliary midwifery and immunizations of children. Patients requiring hospital admission are usually sent to hospitals in Makkah or Jeddah.

Patients are seen and treated by the doctor and nurses from 8:30 to 12:30 in the mornings and from 4:00 to 7:30 in the afternoon each day except Friday. During these times the center is usually crowded and the staff are kept very busy. Home visits are not normally made by the midwife except for serious emergencies and some home confinements. There is no special clinic for particular health needs such as maternity and child health. There is no environmental health activity nor any community health programs.

On average, 130 patients attended the health center per day. Table (14) shows the distribution of 153 diagnoses made among 136 patients who attended the health center in one day. Among the children below the age of 14, the most frequent conditions were upper and middle respiratory tract infections (22/62 = 35 percent) and gasteritis and abdominal pains (19/62 = 31 percent). Adults had a wide range of different conditions. In the age group 15-44 years, nine of 40 diagnoses in men (22 percent) were trauma or musculo-skeletal problems and 11 out of 38 of those in women (29 percent) were gynecological or obstetric.

Table 14. Diagnoses According to Age and Sex for One Day Attendents Khulais Health Center.

Diagnoses	<5 M	<5 F	5-14 M	5-14 F	15-44 M	15-44 F	45 plus M	45 plus F	All Ages M	All Ages F	T
Upper respiratory	3	4	1	4	6	—	—	—	10	8	18
Cough/laryngitis	6	1	3	—	1	1	—	—	10	2	12
Lower respiratory	—	—	—	—	2	—	—	—	2	—	2
Diarrhea/ vomiting	6	3	4	—	3	1	—	—	13	4	17
Abdominal pain	3	1	—	2	1	4	1	—	5	7	12
Cystitis	—	—	—	—	4	—	—	—	4	—	4
Renal colic	—	—	—	—	3	—	—	—	3	—	3
Gynaecological	—	—	—	—	—	8	—	—	—	8	8
Obstetric	—	—	—	—	—	3	—	—	—	3	3
Ears	—	1	—	—	1	—	—	—	1	1	2
Eyes	—		1	2	2	1	1	—	4	3	7
Trauma	1	—	4	—	4	—	—	—	9	—	9
Skin/hair	1	—	1	—	3	1	2	1	7	2	9
Joints							2	—	2	—	2
Backache	—	—	1	1	—	1	—	1	1	3	4
Muscular	—	—	—	—	5	1	—	1	5	2	7
P.U.O.	1	—	—	—	1	—	1	—	3	—	3
Psychiatric	—	—	—	—	1	3	1	—	2	3	5
General weakness	4	—	—	1	2	6	2	—	8	7	15
Dental	—	—	1	—	—	2	—	—	1	2	3
Other	1	—	—	—	1	6	—	—	2	6	8
Total:	26	10	16	10	40	38	8	5	90	63	153*

Patients with more than one diagnosis are included in each relevant diagnostic category. The total diagnoses, therefore, exceeds the total number of patients seen.

Analysis of one day's prescriptions (Table 15) showed that of 288 items dispensed, tonics accounted for nearly one-third of the total. Of the active preparations prescribed, 62 (30 percent) were antibiotics and 49 (24 percent) were antipyretics/analgesics. The most commonly prescribed antibiotics for children were Keflex drops, tetracycline, triple sulphanomide or ampicillin syrup, and for adult were ampicillin capsules or triple sulphanomide tablets. In 10 cases, antibiotic eye ointments (penicillin or sulphanomide) were prescribed.

Table 15. Drugs Prescribed in One Day at Khulais Health Center.

Drug	No. of Prescriptions
Tonics	83
Antibiotics	62
Antipyretics/Analgesics	49
Anti-spasmodic	28
Anti-diarrhea	16
Anti-allergic	14
Anti-tussive	9
Anti-rheumatic	9
Antacid	5
Laxative	4
Others	9
Total	288

Infectious Disease Notifications

Infectious diseases notifications are based on the clinical diagnosis which are rarely confirmed by microbiological or parasitological investigations. The numbers of cases of each disease notified in the previous 15 months are shown in Table 16. Among children, most of the cases were chicken pox and measles, both of which occured in sharp epidemics between March and June. Tuberculosis was notably absent from among the children, but accounted for more than half the notifications in adults. Cases occurred at a steady rate throughout the year and were found equally in men and women. All cases of influenza occurred in the five winter months and three-quarters of the cases of amebic dysentry were concentrated in a two-month period in October and November.

Table 16. Notification of Infectious Diseases.
(January 1976 - March 1977 Inclusive)

| | | Adults | | |
Disease	Children	Male	Female	Total
Amebic Dysentry	5	19	4	28
Chickenpox	43	18	4	65
Influenza	3	40	23	66
Malaria	1	2	0	3
Measles	46	1	0	47
Mumps	2	0	0	2
Pulmonary T.B.	0	103	101	204
Venereal Diseases	0	3	0	3
Total	100	186	132	418

Maternity Services

The recording of births in the district is incomplete and the dates of birth were recorded only for infants born during the last six months before this survey was carried out. Of the 185 births recorded in this period, only 67 (36 percent) had been attended at home by the midwife.

Vaccination

An analysis of recorded vaccinations during the previous 12 months show the following. The age of vaccination was recorded for 297 recipients of their first dose of DPT; about two-thirds of these (201) were over the age of three years old and only 48 were under the age of one year. The number of second doses of triple (DPT) vaccine was less than half the number of first doses and the number of third doses was only about 10 percent of the number of first doses. Only one child was recorded as having a second dose of polio vaccine and none had a third.

If these records reflect the true position, it is clear that the childhood immunization program is not being effectively implemented. Most children are being vaccinated later than is usually recommended, after the ages of greatest danger, and most are not receiving the full courses of vaccination required to give good protection.

Discussion

The salient facts to emerge from this study are: firstly, that the demands of the health center in Khulais are very great; secondly, there is evidence to suggest that the health care provided is in some aspects inappropriate to the needs and is seriously deficient in other respects; and thirdly, that there have been major recent improvements in the standards of equipment available in the center which should enable better medical care to be provided in the future.

The number of patients attending the clinic each day is high in relation to the staff resources, and the length of time which the doctor can spend with each is inevitably very short. This must adversely affect the standards of clinical medicine and leaves the doctor with little, if any, time to spend on the problems of preventive medicine in the district. An investment of time and resources in this direction should pay dividends by reducing the amount of illness which the center must now try to treat.

The range of clinical conditions which patients present at the health center is wide and many of them are either preventable or relatively trivial, as indicated by the high proportion of tonics prescribed. It seems possible that many of the patients now seen by the doctor might be as well managed by a medical assistant or nurse thus allowing the doctor more time for those who need his skills and attention as well as for community health work.

A relatively high proportion of the patients attended were adults under the age of 45 years of age who might be expected to experience lower morbidity rates than children and older adults. This suggests that the health care being given may not be reaching those in greatest medical need possibly because the very old, the infirm and young children have greatest difficulty in getting to the center, particularly over long distances. Another example of a serious deficiency in the services at present is the low proportion of women whose delivery is attended by a qualified midwife, which is likely to have an important effect on the perinatal mortality rate.

The importance of paying greater attention to preventive health services is highlighted by the large number of cases of tuberculosis notified in adults while, if the figures are correct, none was reported in children.

Schistosomiasis which is essentially preventable, is also highly prevalent in the district. Similarly the number of immunizations recorded was relatively small and there was a signal failure to complete courses of primary immunization in young children.

In conclusion, the study of Khulais health center in 1977 indicated that it was not fulfilling its expected role in promoting the health of the community. The health center is not representative of all health centers in the Kingdom, nevertheless it is not much different from other health centers studied in other parts of the country.

Follow-up Report (1984)

A short visit was paid to Khulais in early 1984 to find if any change has occured in the function of the health center. Some changes, from the time of the first visit in 1977 have been observed (Table 17).

The health center is being moved from the old shabby building to a new roomy one. The Faculty of Medicine at King Abdul Aziz University in Jeddah is using the health center in community medicine training for medical students.

Table 17. Expansion of Health Services in Khulais 1977 –– 1984.

	1977	1984
Population served	18,000	33,000
Staff - doctors	1	3
- dentists	--	1
- paramedicals	6	9
Average outpatients per day	130	280*
Outpatients per doctor	130	93

* excluding dental cases.

The health center is still patient oriented. Over a six-month period in 1984, the midwife assisted in 168 deliveries at homes compared to 67 in 1977. Some progress was noted in immunization. Table (18)

Table 18 Immunization in Khulais Over a Period of One Year. (1977 — 1983).

Antigen	Number	Vaccinated
	1977	1983
DPT. 1st dose	465	479
2nd dose	194	433
3rd dose	47	432
Polio: 1st dose	207	479
2nd dose	1	433
3rd dose	0	432
Smallpox	32	––
Cholera	122	––
Typhoid	19	70

The improvement in immunization is mostly due to a better awareness of the people and the new regulation that no birth certificate is issued unless the child completes his vaccination. There is no follow-up of the default cases by the health center.

In Conclusion:

The health center has expanded its services in the last seven years. However, the servies are still directed to those who attend the health center. It is curative oriented. Except for the immunization programs, little community based action is being given in the health center in terms of environmental health, health education, expanded immunization program, community health diagnosis or early detection of diseases. The physicians and their staff (except for birth attendants) are not permitted to visit homes.

This is not different from other health centers studied in the 1980's in the country, namely in Qasim Region (1980) and Turaba Valley (1981).

BIBLIOGRAPHY

1. Bayoumi RA, Omer A, Samuel APW, Saha N. Sebai ZA, Sabaa HMA. Hemoglobin and Erythorocytic Glucose-6-Phosphate Dehydrogenase varients among selected tribes in Western Saudi Arabia. Tropical and Geographical Medicine 1979; 31: 245-252.

2. Miller D, Sebai ZA. Evaluation of the Khulais Health Center in Rural Arabia. In: Mahgoub E. ed Proceedings of Fifth Saudi Medical Meeting. Riyadh: University of Riyadh Press, 1980: 69-80.

3. Saha N, Bayoumi RA, El-Sheikh FS, et al. Some Blood Genetic Markers of Selected Tribes in Saudi Arabia. American Journal of Physical Anthropology; 52: 595 -600.

4. Sebai ZA, Miller DL, Ba'aqeel H. A Study of Three Health Centers in Rural Saudi Arabia. Saudi Medical Journal 1980; 1;4: 197-202.

5. Dacie JV, Lewis SM. Practical Hematology. 5th Ed. London: Churchill Livingstone, 1975.

6. Motulsky AG, Campbell-Kraut JM. Population Genetics of Glucose-6-Phosphate Dehydrogenase Deficiency Red Cell. In: Blumbeg GS. ed. Proceedings of the Conference of Genetic Polymorphisms and Geographic Variation in Disease. New York: Grune-Stratton, 1961: 159-80.

III - TAMNIA

The health status of preschool children reflects the health condition of the commmunity as a whole. It also helps to formulate baseline data for planning, follow-up and evaluation of health programs.

The objective of the community health survey, conducted in the Tamnia villages in the winter of 1979, was to assess the health status of preschool children and interrelated socioeconomic and environmental factors. It was carried out as an education-research project by a team of three staff members from King Saud Faculty of Medicine, two pediatricians from King Faisal Specialist Hospital and 12 medical students in their penultimate year. The project was cosponsored by King Saud University, the Ministry of Health and King Faisal Specialist Hospital.

This section discusses in brief the results of the clinical, anthropometric and laboratory examination of 279 preschool children. It was hoped the results would shed light on certain aspects of the health problems of children, and how they are to be met by the primary health care setup.

Tamnia is a cluster of nine villages on the Sarawat Mountain, Asir Province, in the southwest of Saudi Arabia (Figure 7 p. 32). The villages stretch over an area of five square kilometers at a distance of about 40 kilometers from the city of Abha, the capital of the Asir. The population of Tamnia is 2053, of which 518 are six years or under. The economy of the villagers depends on farming, trading and government employment.

Methodology

Of 518 preschool children a randomly selected sample of 279 children was examined clinically and anthropometrically. Only 257 were investigated by laboratory tests. The sample was drawn randomly from the nine villages. The work was carried out by medical students under the direct supervision of their professors.

1. Clinical examinations: for signs of malnutrition and infection: Conjunctival and corneal xerosis, corneal ulceration, angular stomatitis,

gingivitis, glossitis, nasolabial seborrhea, hair depigmentation, goiter, hepatomegaly, splenomegaly, pyodermia and leishmania scars.

2. Anthropometric measurements: For height, using a wooden measuring board for supine and standing height, and weight, using Salter hanging scales.

3. Laboratory investigations: Blood, stool and urine tests were carried out on 257 preschool children. Twenty percent of the samples were checked for reliability.

The Findings

Clinical and anthropometric measurements:

The age and sex distribution of the 279 children examined clinically and anthropometrically is shown in Table 19.

Table 19. Age and Sex Distribution of 279 Children Surveyed in Tamnia.

Age group in months	Males	Females	Total
1 - 5	12	9	21
6-11	8	12	20
12-23	26	16	42
24 - 35	25	18	43
36 - 47	22	23	45
48 - 59	32	26	58
60 - 72	21	29	50
Total	146	133	279

Except for two infants with marasmus and one infant with rickets, no other clinical signs of drastic malnutrition or vitamin deficieny were seen. Ten children had mild to moderate enlargement of the liver and three children had mild splenic enlargement. In the absence of clinical and laboratory findings of schistosomiasis and malaria, the cause of the enlarged liver is likely to be nutritional.

The heights age and weights for heights were related to the median of the Harvard standard and children were classified as stunted or wasted in their growth according to recommendations for surveys of similar scope and purposes.[1,2,3]

Table 20 presents the distribution of children with deficits in weight-for-height indicating wasting or acute malnutrition and the distribution of children with deficits in height-for-age - indicating stunting or chronic malnutrition.[4] The point prevalence of children with moderate wasting was 2 percent and less than 1 percent of the children were severely wasted. The point of prevalence of the children with moderate stunting was 23 percent, while 4 percent of the children were found to be severely stunted.

Table 20. Degree of Wasting and Stunting of 277 Tamnia Children (In Reference to Havard Standard).

	Percentage of Children			
	Normal	Mild	Moderate	Severe
Degree of Wasting	60	37	2	1
Degree of Stunting	30	43	23	4

Cut-off Points:

Wasting: More than 90 percent normal; 80 - 90 percent mild; 70 - 80 percent moderate; less than 70 percent severe.

Stunting: More than 95 percent normal; 90 - 95 percent mild; 95 - 90 percent moderate; less than 85 percent severe.

The prevalence of wasting is low compared to other areas of Saudi Arabia[5] and other developing countries.[4,6] The relatively high prevalence of moderate stunting among children (23 percent) may imply the presence of past long-term nutritional deprivation of a more subtle nature in combination with chronic and recurrent infectious diseases. The unusual difference between the moderate degrees of stunting and wasting can be explained either by a change over time in quantitative or qualitative food intake, diseases of early childhood or genetic factors.

Figure 12 shows an action diagram based on the estimated degrees of wasting and stunting. It indicates that 28 percent of the preschool children need planned action, in term of better curative and preventive health services.

Figure 12. GRADES OF WASTING AND STUNTING AMONG TAMNIA CHILDREN (0 - 72 MONTHS)

		STUNTING PERCENTAGE OF REFERENCE MEDIAN HEIGHT FOR AGE	
	NORMAL ≥ 95 MILD 90 - 94	MODERATE 85 - 89 SEVERE <85	
NORMAL ≥ 90 MILD 80 - 89	NO ACTION 72%	ACTION 26%	
MODERATE 70 -79 SEVERE <70	ACTION 1.5%	URGENT 0.5%	

(Left axis label: PERCENTAGE OF REFERENCE MEDIAN WEIGHT FOR HEIGHT — WASTING)

Laboratory Tests:

Laboratory findings revealed that a significant number of the children were anemic (Table 21 and Figure 13). Hematological parameters (measured according to Dacie and Lewis[7]) indicated that the anemia, though usually mild, was most often due to nutritional deficiencies or to parasitic infection. The latter relationship is clearly shown in Table 22 and is supported by the albumin/globulin ratio determinations. However, other causes of anemia were found; a case of HbH was diagnosed on electrophoresis, and cases of anemia with microcytic hypochromic cells and normal iron concentration indicated that thalassemia is present in the population of Tamnia. Parents were unfortunately not available for investigation. While no attempt was made to carry out HbA_2 estimation, agar electrophoresis at alkaline pH (Corning 1974[8]) did not demonstrate any values higher than normal. The blood films showed that about 10 percent of the anemic children had megaloblastic anemia, suggestive of Vitamin B_{12} deficiency. No hemoglobin structural abnormalities were identified by hemoglobin electrophoresis.

Protein electrophoresis patterns were consistent with the findings of parasites in the stools, and an increase in the acute phase proteins was also observed in these children.

Table 21. Overall Hemoglobin Mean Values for 257 Preschool Children in Tamnia.

No. of Subjects	Hemoglobin (g/dl)	Mean Values (g/dl)
91	< 11.2	9.4
138	11.2 - 14.8	12.6
28	> 14.8	15.4

Table 22. Mean Hematological Values in Parasite - Infested and Parasite Free Preschool Children in Tamnia.

	Hemoglobin (g/dl)	PCV (%)	RBC (x10 ^{12}/1)	WBC (x10^9/1)
Infested Children	9.9 + 1.0	37.9 + 1.4	3.98 + 0.8	9.6
Non-infested children	13.57 + 1.7	41.8 + 1.6	4.7 + 0.7	8.9

Monoclonal bands were also demonstrated on electrophoresis in three individuals from Al-Yanfa. Three families with G-6-PD deficiency were indentified.

The Tamnia villages are free from malaria. The high prevalence of parasitic infection found in the stools (using Burrows method[9]) is shown in Table 23.

Table 23. Prevalence of Parasitic Diseases in Preschool Children.

Parasite	No. Infested	Prevalence (%)
Ascaris lumbricoides	37	15.7
Hymenolepis nana	25	10.6
Giardia lamblia	22	9.4
Entamorobius vermicularis	3	1.3
Entamoeba histolytica	2	0.9

The most common Blood groups found were A + and O+.

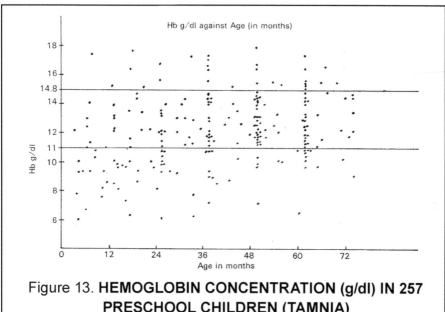

Figure 13. **HEMOGLOBIN CONCENTRATION (g/dl) IN 257 PRESCHOOL CHILDREN (TAMNIA)**

Discussion:

The most striking clinical feature of the preschool children was disturbances in growth. The nutritional problem in Tamnia stems mostly from a lack of awareness on the part of the people of the nutritional values of various foods which are already available in the community. The high incidence of moderate stunting could be due to the synergetic action of pneumonia, diarrhea and malnutrition during early childhood. All that is needed is well directed community-based health care programs, including health education, immunization and nutrition.

The findings of a significant level of anemia and chronic parasitic infections indicate the need for basic laboratory investigations to be available in rural health centers. These tests are cheap and easy to carry out and would contribute considerably to the early diagnosis of health problems in the community.

BIBLIOGRAPHY

1. Waterlow JC, Buzina R, Keller W, Lane JM, Nichaman MZ, Tanner JM. Bulletin of the World Health Organization, 1977; 55: 489 - 98.

2. Miller DC, Nichaman MZ, Lane JM. Bulletin of the World Health Organization, 1977; 55: 79.

3. Report of Joint FAO/UNIFEF/WHO Expert Committee. Methodology of Nutritional Surveillance. WHO Technical Report Series. Geneva, 1976; 593.

4. Waterlow JC. In: Cravioto J, et al. Ed. Early Malnutrition and Mental Development. Uppsala: Almquist and Wikell, 1974.

5. Serenius F, Fougerouse D. Health and Nutritional Status in Rural Saudi Arabia. Saudi Medical Journal, 1981; Suppl. 1: 10.

6. Brink EW, Khan IH, Splitter JL, et al. Bulletin of the World Health Orgnization, 1976; 54: 311 - 18.

7. Dacie JV, Lewis SM. Practical Hematology. 5th ed. London: Churchill Livingstone, 1975.

8. Corning. EEL Agarose Film/Casette Electrophoresis. No. 001 91 146A ed. 1974.

9. Burrows RB. Microscopic Diagnosis of the Parasites of Man. New Haven: Yale University Press, 1965.

IV - QASIM

With modern advancements in medical sciences and technologies, there is an abundance of information so that it is virtually impossible to feed the needed information to the students in the medical schools. Undergraduate education should prepare medical students to be able to educate themselves continuously, think rationally and solve problems in real life situations.

In order to study the impact of socioeconomic and environmental factors on the health of the people, the training of medical students in the community should be complimentary to classroom and hospital teaching. It also provides the students with an opportunity to learn how to organize a health team, generate comprehensive health care and initiate community participation.

In the spring of 1980, the Community Medicine Department of King Saud Faculty of Medicine organized a two-week project in the villages of Ein and Khusaiba (total population of 3,100 inhabitants) in the Qasim Region (Figure 7 Page 29). A team of 18 faculty members and medical specialists from the Ministry of Health, 30 medical students in the prefinal year, and 22 health assistants participated in the project. The objective was to train the medical students in the basic clinical epidemiology and to expose them to community health problems in rural Saudi Arabia.

The team carried out several studies to assess the health situation of the community, including the following:

- A battery of clinical and laboratory tests to screen the health status of young children

- Anthropometric measurements

- Household surveys of socioeconomic status and family nutrition

- Environmental sanitation

- Epidemiology of road accidents

- Evaluation of health services

- Local healers and medicinal plants

The methodology and the findings of the project were published in a monograph by the Saudi Medical Journal.[1] In this chapter we will discuss the following topics:

A. A Profile of the Qasim Region

B. The Field Project, Concept and Methodology

C. The Family Setting

D. Health Status of Preschool Children

E. Primary Health Care

The health manpower will be discussed in Chapter IV.

Profile of the Qasim Region

Area: Approximately 80,000 square kilometers.

Population: Approximately 370,000; 65 percent settled, 20 percent semi-settled, 15 percent nomad.

Cities and Villages: The three main cities are Breida - 120,000 population, Eneiza - 55,000 population, Al Rass - 35,000 population. There are about 600 villages and settlement areas.

Main Occupations: Farming, government employment and trade.

Temperature: Average 24°C (0 - 45°C).

Rainfall: Average 80 mm per year, mainly in winter.

Main Wadi: Al Rumma.

Altitude: 600 meters above sea level.

Agriculture: One of the most cultivated areas in the country. The main products are wheat, dates and vegetables.

Distance from Riyadh: 470 kilometers, asphalted roads.

Hospitals: Three general (Breida, Eneiza, Al Rass), one fever, one tuberculosis. Total beds - 459.

Health Centers: 42 (staffed by physicians).

Dispensaries: 28 (staffed by male nurses).

Number of Physicians: 264 (only two physicians are Saudi).

The Qasim Region is known for its fertile land and abundance of underground water. Agricultural products include cereals (mainly wheat), dates, vegetables and citrus fruits. Part of the product is consumed locally and the remainder distributed to the rest of the Kingdom and exported to the Gulf States.

The inhabitants of Qasim are the descendants of many nomadic tribes. The first settlers came from Etaiba, Bani Tamim, Harb, Shammar, Mutair and Enaza tribes, among others.

The main occupations of the people are trading, farming, government employment and, to a lesser extent, animal husbandry.
Nomadic Bedouins still roam the northeastern part of Qasim. They are, however, settling rapidly, partly because of the drought and partly because settlement life is becoming more comfortable and economically rewarding. Many of the new settlers work in the National Guard, cultivate the land and still keep some of their animals.

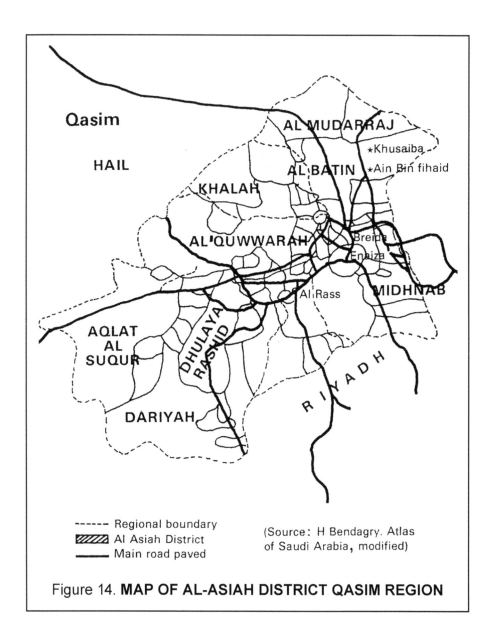

Figure 14. **MAP OF AL-ASIAH DISTRICT QASIM REGION**

The area of cultivated land is rapidly increasing due to the acceleration of Bedouin settlement encouraged by the government. Free land and technical and financial aid are available to the farmers through the Ministry of Agriculture and the agricultural bank. There is even a movement back to the area of young Qasim men who have lived and worked in the large cities such as Riyadh and Dammam. This is somewhat different from the general trend of rapid ubanization observed in the country as a whole.

A noticeable trend also is the appearance of a large number of expatriates from non-traditional nationalities such as Filipinos and South Koreans. The number of expatriates from the Middle East and Pakistan also continues to rise.

Rapid changes are occurring in girl's education in Qasim. The first school for girls in Qasim was opened in 1961 and was faced with great opposition from the people. Now there are about 30 girls schools (primary, intermediate and secondary) and their number is steadily rising. They are all separated from the boys schools. A faculty of women teachers is expected to be opened soon.

A man in Qasim does not object to his daughter studying for a college degree or even working. Almost all the teachers in one village girls school are female Saudis. The father makes only one condition - that his daughter should not come in direct contact with men. In other words, a father can agree to his daughter working as a teacher or social worker if she has contact with women only. Many fathers do not like to see their daughters work as nurses, since this profession would bring them into contact with men.

Learning medicine is, however, different "for a woman doctor can take care of herself." It is little wonder that the enrollment of girls in medical schools in the country is increasing while little interest is shown in nursing.

Al Asiah District

In Al Asiah District (Figure 14) there are 12 villages with a total population of approximately 11,800 (ranging from 200 to 2,700 per village). The district extends over an area of 750 square kilometers. A few nomadic Bedouins still wander on the eastern side herding goats and sheep. Some of the nomads have recently made their homes in settlement areas such as Khusaiba and practice agriculture there.

Although many of the older generation are illiterate, most of the young boys and girls attend school. There are 17 boys schools with a total of 1,356 pupils and 10 girls schools with 811 pupils. Almost all the schools were established during the last two decades.

The economy of Al Asiah does not differ much from that of the rest of the region. In Ain, an old settled community, a man's main occupation is agriculture, trade or government employment, and in many instances his income depends on more than one source. Almost all tradesmen, such as butchers, carpenters, tailors, etc. and manual workers are non-Saudis. Ain is one of the few villages in Qasim where 30 percent of the inhabitants are of Negroid origin. This is because a century ago slaves were imported to this region to help in farming.

In Khusaiba, a newly settled community, the people practice limited agriculture. The main source of income is employment with the National Guard. This takes many of the young adults, sometimes with their families, to cities for several months a year.

In Al Asiah, as in other rural communities in Saudi Arabia, there are very close family and tribal ties. If a tribesman faces a crisis (accident, sickness, death, etc.) all his relatives, neighbors and fellow tribesmen will collectively support him (Furga). Occasionally, needy people visit their relatives or fellow tribesmen working in the cities and ask for financial help (Rafda). About 15 percent of the people are supported by the social security system. This provides SR1,080 per year for the disabled, the aged and widows.

Many changes have occurred over the last decades or so, mostly due to the better income of the people. In the early 1960's, many villagers and Bedouins lived at subsistence level. The main food of a rural family then was rice, bread and tomato sauce. Then in the early 1970's came the era of flourishing economy. This has affected almost all aspects of the people's lives.

Modern health services are available. There are two health centers in Ain and Khusaiba, four dispensaries - in Hunaidel, Al Jeala, Tannoma and Abul Dood - and a general hospital in Breida, 60 kilometers away.

People still occasionally refer to native medicine. Local herbs are readily available in almost every house for day-to-day complaints such as headache, minor fever, constipation or body aches. There is always a "wise old woman" in the neighborhood who is ready to give advice or to carry out some superficial cautery on the heels or around the umbilicus when simple diarrhea or abdominal colic is the problem.

There are half a dozen professional native healers in Al Asiah who handle more serious problems. Bone-setting is a task which everyone in Qasim believes a Bedouin practitioner carries out better than a doctor. Other healers perform cautery or prescribe local herbs in treating problems such as enlarged spleen, jaundice (Al Safari), pleurisy (Jamba), or even cataract. Bleeding (Hejama) is not commonly practiced.

The Field Project, Concept and Methodology

This section will address the educational aspects with the following highlights:

- The reorientation of the faculty towards community-based education

- Community participation

- Student involvement

The Reorientation of the Faculty

I still remember the response of the faculty board in 1975 when we submitted our first proposal to take 20 medical students out to a rural community. The proposal was initially rejected on grounds that the field work would deprive the students of their classes and hospital wards. Finally it was approved with reluctance.

In the following years we organized several field projects and observed a progressive improvement in the attitude of the faculty. For example, our main problem in 1980 was to select only 13 staff members out of 40 or more who wanted to join us.

The case of the consultant **ophthalmologist** is an example of how the attitude of educators could be positively changed simply by exposure. He was asked in 1979 to supervise a group of medical students in surveying eye-health problems in a village. His response: "I am a clinician and interested in my research, not in community medicine or in training the students." We accepted him on his conditions. In 1980 he joined us again and he was a great enthusiast in carrying out a trachoma control program.

The planning phase of the project took several months. Members of various departments in the medical school (medicine, surgery, pediatrics, biochemistry, ophtalmology, ENT and orthopedics) and a number of specialists from the Ministry of Health were solicited to join the project. Several meetings were held to define the objectives of the project, the activities to be undertaken and the timetable. Six teams of students and educators were formed and each team had to prepare its protocol of a specific activity. The protocols were then discussed and adjusted in the light of the general framework of the project.

The point to be emphasized is that it is highly possibly to reorient educators towards innovative concepts of medical education through appropriate learning experiences.

Community Participation

In the planning phase, we selected the Qasim region as the site for the project. We traveled extensively in the region and visited several villages in order to select the local community. One main condition we made in the selection of the community was the readiness of the people to participate actively in the project. This issue was raised and discussed with the sheikhs and leaders of all the villages we visited, and we found that the people were consistently responsive.

The selection of the two villages was based on the appropriate size of population, the presence of a primary school and a health center, the accessibility to the main town in Qasim and, more than anything else, the willingness of the community to participate in the project.

All possible means were employed to ensure that the community felt identified with the project and was responsible for its success. Before the commencement of the project we paid several visits to the two villages and we explained thoroughly and in simple language the purpose of the project - that it is educational for the medical students and the findings will be reported to the health authorities with recommendations for improving the health services. Also, we would treat the sick in collaboration with the local health center. On our visits we were accompanied by authorities from the capital of the region who were also involved in the project planning and implementation.

Several people played an active role; for instance, a group of male teachers in Khusaiba volunteered to map the village (Figure 15) and conduct a demographic survey and a group of female teachers was trained to carry out the household survey. The community provided us with accommodation, food and transportation. Towards the end of the fieldwork, the community was activated to undertake a program of trachoma control, child immunization and health education. Action was to be implemented by school children, under the supervision of their teachers. All the events proved that people are ready to participate actively in their own health programs if adequately oriented.

Student Involvement

Students were active participants in the project. Early in the planning phase the class of 30 students participated in defining the objectives and methodology, communicating with the administration, preparing the budget, purchasing equipment and supplies, and other planning activities. A committee of five students was responsible for coordination.

While in the field, students, besides their assignments in the survey, were responsible for the logistics including housing, transportation, food and communications. They also organized a cleaning day in which the community and our team together cleaned the villages.

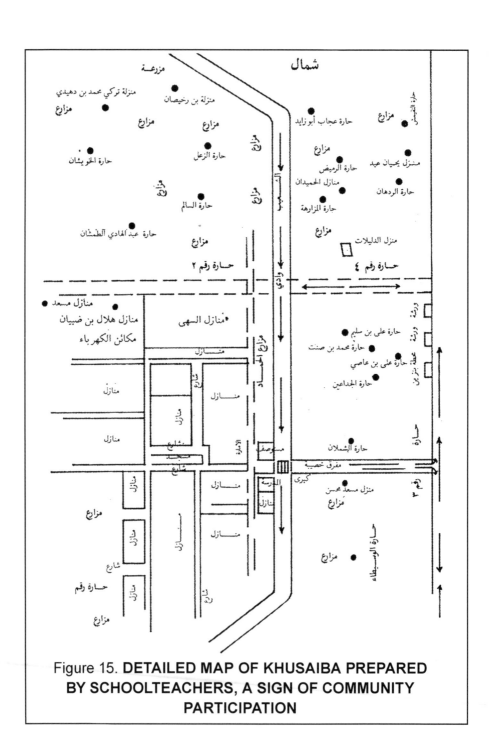

Figure 15. **DETAILED MAP OF KHUSAIBA PREPARED BY SCHOOLTEACHERS, A SIGN OF COMMUNITY PARTICIPATION**

Back in Riyadh, the students, under supervision, analysed the data, documented the results and organized a two-day symposium on the project.

To determine what students had learned most from the project, a questionnaire was distributed among them. Their responses included the following:

- Awareness of health problems in rural Saudi Arabia

- Methodology of a survey

- Planning and conducting a health project

- The value of teamwork

Students can be an excellent planners and organizers if they are given a chance.

The Educational Experience

For both the staff and the students, the educational experience cannot be overemphasized. The project became a topic for group discussions in classes and examinations, a book was published, several papers were presented in scientific meetings and a 16mm documentary film was produced. For many, it was the first exposure to the life in a Saudi village. Leading a simple life, sleeping on the ground in mud houses and sharing food with the people in the village gave us excitement and joy. The morale and spirit of the group was high and the active participation of the people was a real thrill.

Such a short-term experience is not a substitute for a more elaborate program of community-based education. The ultimate goal is to prepare future physicians for a more comprehensive and holistic approach.

The Family Setting

We studied some of the factors within the family setting which may influence the health of the preschool child.

One hundred and nine mothers were interviewed concerning literacy, age of first marriage, number of pregnancies and their outcome and concepts of family planning. The interviews were conducted by four female nurses and social workers from the community who had been trained for the task.

The heads of 198 households were interviewed by four male medical students to record information on various aspects of the family setting. At the same time, informal discussions were held with key informants from both communities.

The Mothers' Perspective

The 109 responding mothers were aged from 15 to 40 years (Table 24). The mean age of mothers from both villages was 23 years.

Table 24. Distribution of Mothers According to Age Group.

Age Group (years)	Ain	Khusaiba	Total
15		1	1
16 - 20	13	6	19
21 - 30	26	27	53
31 - 40	16	20	36
Total	55	54	109

Most of the mothers were illiterate and none had completed primary education. However, almost all the girls of school age were enrolled in the schools of the two villages.

Consanguinity was common. About 65 percent of the mothers were married to a cousin or other relative. Early marriage is the pattern; it usually takes place at the age of 17 years and about 80 percent are married before the age of 20. Very early marriage - before the age of 14 - seldom occurs.

The information from 109 mothers revealed: 540 pregnancies, 520 live births, 27 deaths of children during the first year of life and 17 deaths of children between one and five years of age.

The infant mortality rate (IMR) was estimated at 52 per 1,000 births. This is quite different from other figures of IMR in Saudi Arabia quoted by other authors; 134 in Turaba[2] and 144 in Tamnia.[3] All studies were based on cross-sectional surveys of small non-representative samples of population (including this study). There is a need for a longitudinal prospective study based on a representative sample of population.

The average number of pregnancies was five (ranging from one to 12). Family planning was not commonly practiced. Twenty-nine mothers had some knowledge of contraceptives but none of them admitted using them. However, a new attitude was evident among the young mothers who felt that limiting the number of pregnancies could preserve the mother's health.

In responses to the question "How many more children do you want to have?" 21 mothers wanted no more children, 32 mothers want more boys, four mothers were in favor of girls and 52 mothers had different answers: "as God wishes," "want happiness" and "want health." More mothers were in favor of boys since they provide security in old age and ensure the continuation of the family.

Mothers eat small daily portions of hulba for 40 days after delivery. This they believe, helps in cleaning the womb. Rice is not believed to be a good nutrient for a lactating mother.

Of the 109 mothers, 12 (11 percent) had deliveries in hospital and the other 97 at home. Among the domiciliary deliveries, 85 were assisted either by elderly relatives or by neighbors; only 12 were assisted by a nurse from the health center.

At the time of the survey, 18 mothers were pregnant. None of them received adequate or regular antenatal care.

The mothers were asked about their health complaints in the two weeks before the survey. Out of 109 there were 60 who had complaints including bodyaches (28), headache (11), fever (7), cough (4) and others (10). Of these, 75 percent had received treatment at the health center or the hospital.

The Household-head Perspective

Interviews with 198 heads of households were conducted, 92 from Ain and 106 from Khusaiba. Twenty-eight of the total (14 percent) were black. Thirty-nine (20 percent) had some school education, 93 (47 percent) could read and write although they had no formal schooling and 75 (38 percent) were illiterate. Formal education in Qasim started in the late 1950's and by now practically every boy of school age is enrolled in school.

Family Nutrition

Some differences in family nutrition between the two communities, Khusaiba and Ain, were observed.

In Khusaiba, people breakfast on bread, milk and tea. At lunch time, the main meal for the family is kabsa (rice and meat) which is the staple food. Other alternatives for lunch are margoog or gareesh, all made of flour, meat, tomato sauce and vegetables. Chicken and eggs are not commonly eaten. The evening meal consists of either left-over food from lunch or imported canned food such as cheese, marmalade, cream and butter.

In Khusaiba there is no butcher or baker. The family slaughters a sheep and preserves it in the refrigerator. Each household bakes its own bread. A poor to average income family would reserve the meat for occasions when they have guests - and they have guests frequently. On such occasions, the host family invites neighbors and relatives to share the meal.

On many occasions a complete sheep will be slaughtered, cooked for the guests and laid on a bed of rice. Chicken or goats are not a symbol of hospitality. The food is given first to men who may be joined by grown-up male children - older than six years. The remainder is taken back to the women. The study conducted among nomadic tribes in Turaba in 1967 showed a lag in the physical development of girls, possibly because of the preferential treatment of boys.[4] For many, this generous hospitality is a real burden on the family income (up to 30 percent). Nevertheless, it is part of their heritage.

In Ain, the more settled community, the staple food is still Kabsa but vegetables, fruit, chicken and imported canned foods are part of the dietary pattern. Meat is eaten regularly. Generous parties are given for guests but not on the same scale as in nomadic or recently settled communities.

Feeding Habits of Infants and Children

The newborn baby, soon after birth, is given either water or ghee (Semnah) as a prelactal feed. This is said to lubricate the gut. The child is then breast-fed on demand. Of the 325 preschool children studied, 191 (58.8 percent) were fed by breast milk alone. One hundred and sixteen (35.7 percent) receive supplementary bottle feeding and 18 (5.5 percent) were fed by bottle only. The tendency to use the bottle, alone or as a supplement to breast-feeding was more common in Ain than in Khusaiba, especially among young mothers. Twelve varieties of powdered milk are available on the local market.

In a study conducted in 1967 in villages and nomadic communities in Turaba, Saudi Arabia, it was found that the percentage of children below the age of two years who received powdered milk, either supplementary to breast feeding or alone, was 32 percent in the village and four percent in the nomadic communities.[5] This compares with 41.2 percent in this study. Apparently the practice of bottle feeding has increased in Saudi Arabia as is the case in many other developing countries. It has become a status symbol of modernization and sophistication.

Most of the mothers were ignorant about the methods of preparation and sterilization of the bottle and most of them used a single bottle all the time. The amount of powdered milk used for the feed was, in general much less than that indicated. Until recently the practice of bottle feeding was encouraged by physicians who took care to distribute samples of powdered milk among the mothers. This, however, has recently been forbidden by the health authorities and a campaign against artificial feeding has been launched by the Ministry of Health.

The method of introducing babies to solid foods is the same in both villages. A baby of five months is given sips of orange juice or other available fluids. Occasionally the child is given semi-solid food and the mother may masticate it beforehand. When the child reaches eight to nine months of age, he is welcomed to share the family food. The reason for delaying the introduction to solid foods is that "it causes diarrhea in young babies."

Failure of people to give enough supplementary food is one of the main causes of malnutrition in developing countries.[6] In our study, both the quantity and quality of the supplementary food given before the end of the first year were inadequate. People need to know how to use locally available foods such as peas, beans, rice, vegetables and eggs to supplement child feeding.

A child is weaned on reaching his second birthday. Many Muslim communities adhere to this date of weaning for religious beliefs (Holy Qur'an: chapters Cow, Al Ahgaf and Luqman). A mother will wean her child earlier if she becomes pregnant, for "a pregnant mother's milk can harm the child," or if the mother or child becomes sick. The average weaning age in these villages was 12.5 months. Eleven percent of the mothers continued to breast-feed their children for more than two years. This is done mainly for the precious male child. Seventy-five percent of children were weaned suddenly and 25 percent gradually. Methods used for weaning included painting the nipples with a noxious substance such as red pepper, frightening the child, separating him from his mother for a while, or bribing him. The people realize that weaning can cause emotional trauma.

Economic Status

It is difficult to obtain reliable data about family income. From earlier experiences in the field, heads of families were found to underestimate their income, hoping for some financial aid from the government. Several methods were used in our study to estimate the economic status.

Of the heads of households, 43 percent were in government services, 32 percent were tradesmen, 14 percent were farmers, 7.5 percent had other jobs and 3.5 percent were unemployed. Most of the respondents had more than one source of income. Many of the farmers employed expatriate laborers.

Another approach was to ask our key informants, two from each community, to estimate the income of respondents. Three categories were used: (1) Low income, less than SR1,000 per month. (2) Moderate income, SR1,000 to 2,000 per month. (3) High income, more than SR2,000 per month.

It was estimated that 42 percent of households were in the low income group, 35 percent in the moderate income group and 23 percent in the high income group.

One has to consider, however, that the key informants might not be aware of the actual income of their neighbors. Besides, these figures still mean very little for no information was obtained on how the income was spent, i.e. how much of it goes towards food, clothes, accommodation and other commodities.

Collecting information about the tangible wealth of the household was another method used. Out of 198 households, 80 percent had either a refrigerator (equal to 15 days wages for a normal worker), or a car or pick-up truck (equal to about four months wages), or both. About 79 percent own their own houses through interest-free bank loans.

In our sample there was no significant difference in the education or economic status between the heads of households in the two communities, or between the two races, white and black.

Marriage Customs

Girls put on the veil by the age of 12 years and ordinarily marry at the age of 16 or 17, while men marry between the ages of 20 and 25 years. The marriage is arranged by the family of the prospective bridegroom; his mother or a female relative will choose the bride. The social status of the bride or bridegrooms's family is mainly determined by the wisdom and generosity of the head of the family rather than by his wealth.

A major problem is the great expenses of marriage ceremonies which can easily cost SR80,000 to SR100,000. It is hardly surprising that it is beyond the capacity of many young men unless they are supported by the family or by fellow tribesmen.

The most favored bridegroom is the relative of the bride, particularly a cousin on the father's side. This is especially the case in Khusaiba. The next most favored is someone from the tribe. Some trades are held in such contempt that no tribesman would give the hand of his daughter to a butcher, a baker, a barber, a carpenter or a tailor. Intermarriage between a white woman and a Negro is not known.

Polygamy, allowed in Islam but conditional on the equal treatment of wives, is practiced. It is limited, however, to the older generation. Young and educated men rarely marry more than one wife for a combination of economic and social reasons. "Life is more comfortable and easier with one wife," said a young Qasimi man. Premarital and extramarital sexual relations are strongly prohibited by Islamic Law and are never heard of in rural communities.

A husband may divorce his wife. However, a wife can claim a divorce case of suffering. No reliable statistics exist about the rate of divorce in Qasim, however, family ties and traditions apparently help in stabilizing marital life.

The Population Structure in Khusaiba

A group of four teachers in the boys school in Khusaiba undertook the population survey of Khusaiba village during the preparatory stage of the study. A map of the village was made and serial numbers were painted on the doors of the houses. An information sheet about each household was then completed, this included the name, sex and age of each member of the household. Table 25 shows the population structure of the village. It is more or less a typical structure of a developing country, with 33 percent of the population less than 10 years of age and only four percent of the population aged 60 years or more.

It is not always possible to obtain exact ages from villagers and one has to allow for 10 percent plus or minus the reported age.

Table 25. Khusaiba: Distribution of Population According to Age and Sex.

Age group (Years)	Males	Females	Total	%
0 - 4	55	80	135	17.8
5 - 9	65	53	118	15.5
10- 19	98	68	166	21.8
20 - 29	41	47	88	11.6
30 - 39	54	47	101	13.3
40 - 49	40	33	73	9.6
50 - 59	38	9	47	6.2
60 - 69	22	1	23	3.0
70+	9	—	9	1.2
Total	422	328	760	

Table 26 shows the distribution of Khusaiba people according to the number in the household. There are 760 persons living in 155 houses, an average of 4.9 persons per household. There are 13 vacant houses. The median and the mode are both around the 5.5 figure. This is somewhat different from the extended family which is usually indicated when one talks about an Arab family.

Table 26. Khusaiba: Distribution of Population According to the Number of Individuals Per Household.

No. per Household	No. of Households	Total	%
1	51	51	6.7
2	7	14	1.8
3	7	21	2.8
4	11	44	5.8
5	14	70	9.2
6	15	90	11.8
7	12	84	11.1
8	10	80	10.5
9	10	90	11.8
10+	18	216	28.4
Total	155	760	100.0

Health Status of Preschool Children

A complete census of the population in the two villages was carried out by local school teachers. All families with children under five years of age were included in the study.

Children were examined, with particular emphasis on signs of malnutrition and infectious diseases. Height was measured by Nivotoise tape fixed to the wall and by infantometers. Salter's scales and CMS platform scales were used for weighing. The past history of illnesses and immunization were elicited by interviewing mothers at home. The work was done by pretrained medical students and female nurses under direct supervision.

Data collected on 337 children was analyzed. The age and sex distribution of these children is shown in Table 27. Very few children had birth certificates and few of the mothers knew the exact ages of their children. The problem was overcome by using a local calendar of events.

Table 27. Age and Sex Distribution of 337 Preschool Children.

Age Group (months)	Males	Females	Total
0 -	3	3	6
1 - 5	8	13	21
6-12	29	27	56
13 - 24	40	34	74
25 - 36	37	36	73
37 - 48	30	36	66
49 - 60	17	24	41
Total	164	173	337

History of Morbidity

The incidence of selected common childhood illnesses among the 337 children studied in the month preceding the survey (January 1980) was as follows: 191 (56.7 percent) of the children had fever; 206 (61.1 percent) had cough; 90 (26.7 percent) had diarrhea; and 109 (32.3 percent) had conjunctivitis.

Malnutrition and infections are among the main factors affecting the health of children, particularly of preschool age. The relative high figure given for fever and respiratory tract infections is possibly due to the cold weather in January. Another explanation for the high reporting of fever is that the mother will describe any perceived warmth of the skin of her child as a fever. A thermometer is never used.

A history of measles was given for only 117 children (34.7 percent). Only 17 of these had measles before the age of two years. Morley[7] found that one-third of the children in Africa and the Middle East got measles before the age of one year.

People are aware of the clinical picture of measles (Hasbah). They know that it is contagious and they prohibit their children from visiting an active case. Failure to have the rash is considered a bad sign and hence its appearance is encouraged by giving the child a black pepper solution. It the rash fails to appear by the seventh day, the child is cauterized round the neck. Children are not prohibited from eating any particular food during the measles as is the custom in other parts of the world.[8,9]

Forty children (12 percent) had a history of whooping cough (Shihaig). It is treated locally by honey and cautery and old people recommend drinking the milk of a white donkey as a remedy!

History of Immunization

Table 28 shows the history of vaccination. The relatively high figure for polio vaccinations was due to a recent crash immunization program launched by the regional health services. No reliable history of the exact age of receiving immunization could be revealed in most cases.

Table 28. History of Vaccination of 307 Children.

Vaccine	Children No.	Vaccinated %
Poliomylitis	173	51.3
DPT	73	21.7
BCG	18	5.3
Measles	36	10.7
Not defined	37	11.0

Clinical Examination

Only three cases of severe protein energy malnutrition were diagnosed clinically and confirmed by anthropometry. Two were marasmic and the third had kwashiorker. Three cases of rickets were seen. It is worth noting that rickets is not a rare problem in Qasim and a relatively high prevalence of rickets in central Saudi Arabia has been reported by Idrissy.[10] Signs of other vitamin deficiencies were rare. Not a single case of vitamin A deficiency was seen and only two had angular stomatitis.

Three anthropometric indices —— weight for age, weight for height and height for age - were used to assess the nutritional status of children. Harvard medians[11] were taken as standards and all results are presented as a percentage of the standard. The Gomez Classification[12] was used for weight for age.

Classifications as suggested by Waterlow & Rutishauser[13] and Waterlow[14] were used for the other two indices. A child was considered wasted if weight for height was less than 90 percent of the standard and stunted if height for age was less than 95 percent of the standard.

1. Weight for age: Table 29 shows the weight for age among all surveyed children and in each age group. Only 39.2 percent had normal weight for age, 0.9 percent had severe, 14.5 percent moderate and 45.4 percent mild malnutrition. It was noticed that there was a marked drop in the percentage of normal children after the first year.

2. Weight for height: Table 30 shows the percentage distribution of weight for height among children under the study; 76.3 percent had normal weight for height (i.e. not wasted) whereas 19.8 percent had mild wasting, 3.3 percent moderate wasting and 0.6 percent severe wasting.

3. Height for age: Table 31 shows the percentage distribution of grades of stunting among the children: only 39.1 percent had normal height for age.

4. Table 32 shows the percentage of wasted and stunted children among each age group. Wasting was most common among the 12 and 23 months age group and the percentage of stunted children increased progressively with age.

5. Table 33 shows the percentage distribution of wasting and stunting when both forms of malnutrition were combined. Only 31.2 percent were within normal limits, whereas the rest had either one or both forms of malnutrition in various degrees.

6. In order to device a program of action, the results shown in Table 33 have been classified into four groups and presented in Figure 16, as suggested by Waterlow. Here the top left corner (82.8 percent) represents the 'normal group' who need no action. The bottom right corner represents those who are malnourished and who needed urgent treatment, e.g. hospitalization. The 16.3 percent in the bottom left and top right corners give an indication for some form of action at the community level.

Table 29. Weight For Age: Percentage Distribution of 337 Children by Gomez i Classification (12).

Age Group (months)	Normal nutrition	Percentage of Children with Malnutrition		
		Mild	Moderate	Severe
	(>90%)	(76-90%)	(65-75%)	(<60%)
0 - 5	53	26.5	20.5	--
6 - 11	47.3	38.9	11.1	2.7
12 - 23	37.5	40.6	21.9	--
24 - 35	38.4	53.4	8.2	--
36 - 47	38.8	46.8	11.3	3.1
48 - 60	30	51.4	18.6	--
Total	39.2	45.4	14.5	0.9

Table 30. Weight for Height: Percentage Distribution of 337 Children According to Grades of Wasting.

Grade of Wasting	Percentage of Children
Normal (>90%)	76.3
Mild (80 - 90%)	19.8
Moderate (70 - 79%)	3.3
Severe (<70%)	0.6

Table 31. Height for Age: Percentage Distribution of 337 Children According to Grade of Stunting.

Grade of Stunting	Percentage of Children
Normal (>95%)	39.1
Mild (90 - 95%)	46.3
Moderate (80 - 90%)	11.9
Severe (<80%)	2.7

Table 32. Percentage Distribution of Wasted and Stunted Children Among 337 Children by Age Group.

Age Group (months)	Wasting	Stunting
0 - 5	31	28.2
6 - 11	23.5	52.8
12 - 23	36	57.8
24 - 35	16.4	67.1
36 - 47	19.7	66.1
48 - 60	20.0	71.4

Table 33. Childreh Classified According to Grade of Wasting and Stunting (Percentages).

Grade of Stunting	Grade of Wasting			
	Normal	Mild	Moderate	Severe
Normal	31.2	6.3	1.2	0.3
Mild	37	8.3	2	0
Moderate	8	3	0	0
Severe	0.9	0.9	0.6	0.3

If, as suggested by Waterlow & Rutishauser and Waterlow, children are divided into priority and action groups, then 0.9 percent of Al Asiah children needed urgent action and 16.3 percent needed action by the community. These figures are comparatively lower than the figure of two percent and 27 percent respectively given from the study in the Tamnia region of southwest Saudi Arabia.[15]

Health Services

We studied the function of the two health centers in Ain and Khusaiba. They are not a representative case but evidence suggests that they are not different from others in Saudi Arabia.[16,17]

Each of the two health centers under study is situated in a rented mud house. The 10 rooms in each center are used for clinics, a pharmacy, dressing rooms and storage. Two rooms are kept as the residence for the female nurses. In Ain there is a small laboratory which is not functioning at present. The health services in the two centers are based on outpatient care with very few services extended to the community.

Figure 16. **GRADES OF WASTING AND STUNTING AMONG QASIM CHILDREN (0 - 72 MONTHS)**

GRADE OF WASTING	GRADE OF STUNTING	
	NORMAL + MILD	MODERATE + SERVICE
NORMAL + MILD	NO ACTION 82.8 %	ACTION 3.5%
MODERATE + SEVERE	ACTION 12.8%	URGENT 0.9%

Each health center is staffed by two physicians (a husband and wife), two nurses and a pharmacy assistant. The two physicians working in Khusaiba are from Bangladesh, while the rest of the personnel in the two centers are from Arab countries (mainly Egypt). The only Saudi is a male nurse in Ain.

The four physicians in the two health centers are general practitioners who graduated around 1970. Their period of stay in the country varies from one to five years. Each of the other health personnel has a basic education of nine to 12 years, plus two to three years training. The Saudi nurse has only primary school education and no formal training.

The physicians in charge of the health centers refer directly to the regional director of health services in Qasim. Two or three times a year an inspector from the regional office visits the health centers.

The health services rendered by the two health centers will be discussed under two headings, curative and preventive services.

Curative Services

Table 34 shows the age and sex distribution of those who attended the two health centers over a period of 15 working days. The average number of daily attendances is 90 in Ain and 68 in Khusaiba. In summer the rate of attendance increases by 20 percent. On average 80 percent of those attending are Saudis.

Although the two health centers serve 12 rural communities in an area of about 750 square kilometers, 66 percent of the people attending the center in Ain and 54 percent in Khusaiba come from within a range of five kilometers. The under-12 age group accounts for 37 percent of attendances, which is low in a community where children constitute half the population. In general there are fewer females than males. It is likely that health services are most used by male adults.

The time spent by the physician in seeing his patients was observed and recorded. On average the physician in Ain spent 50 minutes seeing 21 patients (2.4 minutes per patient) and the physician in Khusaiba spent 25.6 minutes attending 17 patients (1.5 minutes per patient). On average, the physicians spent two minutes per patient.

Further analysis of the time spent by the male physician in Ain shows that on average he spends 0.6 minutes for history taking 1.3 minutes for physical examination and 0.5 minutes for prescription writing and guidance of the patient.

Table 34. Number of Outpatients Attending Ain and Khusaiba Health Centers in 15 Days.

	Age Groups				
	0 - 12 yrs		> 12 years		
	Male	Female	Male	Female	Total
Ain	245	202	459	443	1,349
Khusaiba	214	216	336	258	1,024
Total	459	418	795	701	2,373

Forty-four patients (16 male and 28 female) were interviewed after they had been seen by one physician, Of these 91 percent could not state the diagnosis of their ailments - they only mentioned their complaints - and 52 percent did not know how to use the prescribed medicine properly.

Table 35 shows the diagnosis of patients who visited the two health centers over 15 days, as recorded in the physician's book. Diagnosis is made on the basis of the patient's complaint and is recorded in general terms such as disease of the skin, eye, ear, kidney, etc. There is a lack of precision in recording: for example, "conjunctivitis" in Ain is recorded as "eye disease" in Khusaiba.

The ratio of Ain to Khusaiba attendents is almost equal (1:3:1). One would not expect much difference in age and sex distribution or in specific health problems recorded at the two health centers, since the two communities differ little in their health problems and population pattern. But in fact the recordings present a different picture.

Table 35. Diagnosis of Cases Attending the Two Centers in 15 Days (2,373 Cases).

	No. of Patients	
Diagnosis	**Ain**	**Khusaiba**
Common cold	63	224
Tonsillitis	85	79
Diarrhea	96	68
Rheumatism	36	185
Diseases of the skin	100	77
Bronchitis	293	
Conjunctivitis	212	
Moniliasis	43	
Colic	76	
Gastritis, hyperacidity	150	

General weakness	61	
Measles	2	
Dysentry	89	
Hypertension	9	
Pneumonia		15
Disease of the ear		42
Disease of the eye		111
Disease of the tooth		28
Disease of the kidney		8
Bronchial asthma		8
Communicable diseases		2
Chest pain		25
Others	34	152
Total	1,349	1,024

There are many diseases which are recorded in one health center but not the other, e.g. moniliasis, gastritis, general weakness and diseases of the ear, eye, kidney, etc.

Table 36 shows the drugs prescribed in the two health centers over 15 days. No common pattern exists between the two centers; whereas 5.5 items per patient were dispensed in Ain, and 2.5 dispensed in Khusaiba. Items such as tonics and vitamins, antispasmodics and antitussives were dispensed with wide differences between the two centers.

In Ain, out of each 10 patients, nine received antibiotics and/or tonics, vitamins or iron. In Khusaiba, out of each 10 patients, eight received antibiotics and/or tonics, vitamins and iron. These figures reflect unjustifiable over-prescription of drugs.

The differences in the number of drugs dispensed per patient in the two health centers (5.5 items in Ain and 2.5 items in Khusaiba) evidently arises from differences in the physicians' attitudes, their submissiveness to the people's demands and the availability of drugs. This is in addition to the lack of supervision and control. The large number of items dispensed for each patient is an observed pattern of practice among many physicians in the country. Antibiotics, in the form of chloramphenicol, tetracycline, penicillin and septrin were prescribed indiscriminantly and in large quantities. Considering the short examination time, the lack of laboratory facilities for proper diagnosis and sensitivity testing, and the patients' ignorance of the proper use of drugs, we can perceive the possible hazards of indiscriminant prescription of such drugs.

Preventive Services

Preventive and promotive services expected from the primary health care unit in such a community can include health education, maternal and child health care, environmental sanitation, preventive dental care, nutritional programs and recording of statistics. None of these activities is adequately carried out.

The vaccination records are incomplete in the two health centers. From a study on the number of children vaccinated in the area it was evident that less than 7 percent of the preschool children have received complete coverage of polio and triple vaccines.

The physician is prohibited from visiting the patients in their homes. Male physicians are not permitted by the Ministry of Health to carry out vaginal examinations. This task is left for the female practitioner or the specialists in the hospitals.

The only home visits made by the female nurses in the two centers are to attend mothers at birth. The 12 pregnant mothers who attended the Khusaiba health center in one week received medicines for their present complaints. No antenatal or postnatal program is carried out in either of the two centers. no other health services are carried out by the two health centers.

Table 36. Drugs Prescribed in the Two Centers in 15 Days.

Drug	Ain No.	%	Khusaiba No.	%
Antibiotics	1222	16.4	458	17.3
Sulpha	103	1.4	35	1.3
Tonics & Vitamins	1164	15.7	208	7.9
Iron	230	3.1	161	6.1
Antispasmodic	407	5.5	6	0.2
Analgesic	638	8.6	378	14.3
Antidiarrheal	337	4.5	16	0.6
Antitussive	762	10.2	32	1.2
Antacid	291	3.9	191	7.2
Antiallergic	260	3.5	141	5.3
Bronchodilator	147	2.0	9	0.3
Sedative	11	0.1	79	3.0
Eye drops	317	4.2	40	1.5
Ear drops	170	2.3	43	1.6
Others	1401	18.8	851	32.1
Total	7460	100.0	2648	100.0

A simple analysis of the work of the health centers shows that on average, the four physicians see a total of 158 patients a day, with an average of two minutes per patient. This is equal to 1.3 hours of each physician's time. It is evident that the procedure cannot have much effect on the health of the individual or the community.

If we assume that each physician spends two hours on administrative work in addition to the 1.3 hours spent on clinical work, he or she will be left with about 4.5 hours free time per day (eight working hours per day for five and a half working days per week). The same could be applied to the rest of the 10 health personnel working in the two health centers. A simple calculation indicates that total free time is 45 hours per day or 900 hours per month, ample time to operate a wide range spectrum of promotive health activities in the communities.

None of the staff in the two centers has participatd in a continuing education program or attended a medical conference, with the exception of one of the physicians who attended a seven-day seminar on "war medicine." None of the physicians receives medical journals or keeps a library in the clinic. They all feel the need for continuing medical attention.

The physicians in the health centers have their own demands such as opportunities for continuing education, adequate financial and administrative authority and a recognition of their requests for needed drugs and medical supplies.

Follow-up Report (1981)

A two-day visit was paid to Al Asiah area nine months after the completion of the study to see if any change in the health services had occurred in the two communities.

Some definite improvements were observed in Ain village. After we had left Qasim, the health center personnel moved from the old rented building to the new building which we had occupied during the time of the project. The spacious building accommodated an X-ray machine, a small laboratory, a dental clinic and 10 maternity care and emergency beds. More personnel were required to run the service.

The number of deliveries conducted by the two nurses/midwives in the center increased from three per month to 25 per month. About 15 per month were conducted in the center and the rest at home. The diagnostic capability of the two physicians in the center is believed to have improved because of the laboratory and X-ray facilities.

The recent recruitment of a well trained-Arabic speaking health officer has another positive influence. Each newborn child in Ain now has an immunization record and a well maintained system of follow-up is being initiated. People are aware of the importance of immunization for their children. More than 50,000 tetracycline eye ointment tubes and 20,000 bottles of sulpha eyedrops were distributed among the people of Al Asiah to use in the family care system campaign against trachoma. Unfortunately no records of their actual usage are being kept.

The progress we observed in Ain village could be due to a combination of factors almost all of which, we believe, came about as a result of the project:

1. The demonstration to the physicians and their staff of the practicality of and need for delivering some aspects of preventive health services to the community.

2. The orientation of the people to their actual needs through health education programs and their actual participation in the project.

3. The transfer of the health center from the old rented building to a well designed building established for the purpose and with sufficient space, equipment and staff housing.

4. The recruitment of a well trained, Arabic speaking health officer for the health center, who has initiated immunization and sanitation programs.

In Khusaiba village we did not observe much change in the health-center activities, with one exception - the increased number of people demanding vaccination. There are, however, no accurate records or follow-up systems. The main differences between Ain and Khusaiba is that in Khusaiba the health center remained in the old mud house, while in Ain the center occupied the new building.

Conclusion:

One needs little imagination to visualize the possible effects of primary health care on the people's state of health if available human resources were efficiently and effectively utilized. This could only be done if the health personnel were well trained, adequately oriented towards their actual role in the community, and capable of activating people to participate in health programs. In brief, health services in such rural communities are being influenced more than anything else by the medical education received by the physicians and health personnel.

It is hoped that the Ministry of Health and the regional health office in Qasim will make a careful study of the changes which have occurred in the health services of Ain village and use this information to reorganize the current system of primary health care.

No doubt the new trends of the Ministry of Health in the decentralization of authority, regionalization of the health services, concern for health manpower development programs and more coordination with the faculties of medicine will lead to an improvement of health services systems in the foreseeable future.

BIBLIOGRAPHY

1. Sebai ZA. ed. Community Health in Saudi Arabia. A Profile of Two Villages in Qasim Region. Saudi Medical Journal 1982; Monograph No. 1.

2. Sebai ZA. The Health of the Family in a Changing Arabia: A Case Study of Primary Health Care. 3rd ed. Jeddah: Tihama Publications, 1983: 80.

3. Serenius F, Fourgerouse D. Health and Nutritional Status in Rural Saudi Arabia. Saudi Medical Journal 1981; 2 (Suppl. 1): 10.

4. Sebai ZA. The Health of the Family in a Changing Arabia: A Case Study of Primary Health Care. 3rd ed. Jeddah: Tihama Publications, 1983: 85.

5. Ibid. p. 68.

6. Jelliffe BD. The Assessment of the Nutritional Status of the Community. In: WHO Monograph Series No. 53. Geneva: WHO, 1966.

7. Morley D. Transaction of the Royal Society of Tropical Medicine and Hygiene, 1978; 72:433.

8. Ebrahim GJ. Breast Feeding: The Biological Option. London: MacMillan, 1978.

9. Sebai ZA. The Health of the Family in a Changing Arabia: A Case Study of Primary Health Care. 3rd ed. Jeddah: Tihama Publications, 1983: 108.

10. Idrissey ATH. In: Mahgoub ES, et al., eds. Proceedings of the 5th Saudi Medical Meeting, Riyadh, 1980. Riyadh: College of Medicine, University of Riyadh, 1981:409.

11. Stuart HC, Stevenson SS. In: Nelson WE, ed. Textbook of Paediatrics. 11th ed. Philadelphia: Saunders, 1979:12.

12. Gomez F, Ramos G, Frenk S, et al. Journal of Tropical Paediatrics 1956; 2: 77.

13. Waterlow JC, Rutishauser IHE. In: Cravioto J, et al., ed Early Malnutrition and Mental Development. Symposium of the Swedish Nutrition Foundation. Stockholm: Almquist & Wiksell, 1974: 12: 13.

14. Waterlow JC. In: Beaton GH, Bengoa JM, eds. Nutrition and Preventive Medicine. WHO Monograph Series No. 62. Geneva: WHO, 1976: 530.

15. Sebai ZA, El'-Hamza MAF, Serenius F. Health Profile of Preschool Children in Tamnia Villages, Saudi Arabia. Saudi Medical Journal 1981; 2 (Suppl. 1): 68.

16. Sebai ZA, Miller DL, Ba'aqeel H. A Study of Three Health Centers in Rural Saudi Arabia. Saudi Medical Journal 1980; 1: 197.

17. Miller DL, Sebai ZA. Evaluation of the Khulais Health Center in Rural Arabia. In: Mahgoub ES, et al., eds. Proceedings of the 5th Saudi Medical Meeting, Riyadh, 1980. Riyadh: College of Medicine, University of Riyadh, 1981: 69-80.

Chapter IV

SELECTED HEALTH PROBLEMS

Endemic Syphilis
Cholera
Leishmaniasis
Filariasis
Leprosy
Hemaglobinopathies

The health problems presented in this chapter are not selected because of their importance or magnitude, but rather because they were the subject of field surveys conducted by the author and his colleagues. Volume Two of this book will cover a wide spectrum of health problems in Saudi Arabia.

Endemic Syphilis (Bejel)
In A Bedouin Community

This section reports the results and interpretations of a Fluorescent Treponema Antibody (FTA) test study among Bedouins which was part of a comprehensive study conducted in Turaba in western Saudi Arabia in 1967 (see Figure 8).

The objectives of the complete study were to assess general health conditions and interrelated socioeconomic and environmental factors in three communities; settled, semi-settled and nomadic.

The Disease

Endemic syphilis (Bejel) is a chronic inflammatory disease caused by Treponema Pallidum. In the early stages, the disease is characterized by infectious mucocutaneous lesions resembling those of secondary syphilis. After a latent period of undetermined time, other manifestations may appear affecting the skin and long bone. Lesions of the cardiovascular or central nervous system are very rare and congenital transmission of the disease is also extremely rare.

Little has been written about endemic syphilis. In literature, it has been referred to as the disease of the Bedouin, transmitted by direct and indirect contact, possibly through common eating and drinking utensils.[1,2,3] Hudson[4] described the disease as a "contagious, non-veneral, innocent syphilis of Bedouin children." Guthe mentioned Saudi Arabia as one of the "islands" of endemic syphilis in the Mediterranean region.

The first published survey on endemic syphilis in Saudi Arabia was in 1954 and was carried out by a team from the World Health Organization.[5] In the report, recommendations for control were given but no organized action has been taken.

The disease is not known in the western hemisphere. The few cases reported (1968) in Vienna were found among the residents of a crowded asylum.[6]

Material and Methods

A total of 314 households in the three communities of Turaba were selected for the study. These included 87 settled, 121 semi-settled and 105 nomadic households.

Interviews, formal and informal, were held with the heads of households and their wives to cover demography, and histories of morbidity and mortality. The interviewees were asked about their opinions on the most prevalent disease in their communities, their causes and treatments.

The original plan was to draw blood from all children in the study, and from adults who accompanied them to the health center for multi-screening purposes. In the first two weeks of the study 107 blood samples were collected, with much difficulty. The people of Turaba strongly objected the procedure. They, like most Arabs, relate blood to strength, vitality and potency. Rumors began to spread that we were using the power in the blood by adding it to the tea which we frequently drank in the field. Some thought that we were selling the blood to city merchants and others were convinced that we were analysing the blood simply to select their children for the army when they came of age. By the second week we felt that insistence on getting venous from the participants would jeopardize the whole study.

At the end of the study period venous blood was drawn from nine adult male and female Bedouins who came to the health center complaining of Shijar (Bejel). The main complaints were general aching of the body, tiredness, and a history of skin eruptions of undetermined duration.

The venous blood samples of 10 cc each, were drawn by vacutaner syringes. A few drops were used for a malaria smear and an estimate of hemoglobin content, the rest was centrifuged the same day. Sera were separated and kept in a small sterilized plastic vials in a butane gas refrigerator.

Specimens were given serial numbers, then transported in dry ice by plane to the Center for Disease Control in Atlanta, Georgia, for bacteriological and virological studies. FTA tests were carried out on all samples. Due to the lack of sufficient amount of sera, a Venereal Disease Research Laboratory (VDRL) test was run on only 82 samples.

The FTA results were matched with recorded clinical examinations and histories.

Results

Since there is no statistically significant difference in the result of the FTA study between the nomadic and semi-nomadic communities, the data from the two groups will be presented under one category, Bedouins. Table 1 shows the results of FTA test on the separated sera of 107 participants.

Table 1. Prevalence of Seropositive Reaction from the FTA Test for Treponema, by Age Group.

Community	Age in years		Positive	
		Respondents	No.	%
Settled	0 - 4	13	--	--
	5 - 19	16	1	6
	20+	20	5	25
Bedouins	0 - 4	19	4	22
	5 - 19	8	2	25
	20+	31	6	20

The four children in the under four years age group with positive serological findings were nomads. Two of them were brothers, three and four years old, living in a nuclear family. The mother had no history of abortion, stillbirth or death of any children.

The other two children showing positive results were one-year-old and four-year-old females. They were also living in small nuclear families in two separate nomadic areas. The mother of one of them was 29 years old. She had six pregnancies and one abortion. The other mother, 35 years old, had three pregnancies and one stillborn fetus.

None of the four children had any specific complaint nor were there any clinical findings of congenital stigmata. These facts indicate acquired rather than congenital syphilis.

Seven out of nine symptomatic adults who had venous blood drawn had positive FTA tests. These were not included in Table 1.

Bejel is well known by the general public in Saudi Arabia under different names such as shijar, mabrouk and infrangi. A Bedouin comes to the health center and tells the doctor "I have shijar," describing his complaints as general bodyache, fatigue, and a history of skin eruptions.

The formal close-ended questionnaire of the 133 heads of households revealed the opinion that the most prevalent diseases in Turaba were whooping cough and measles (72 percent), aching pains (66 percent), shijar (33 percent), diarrhea and fever (14 percent) and tuberculosis (10 percent).

When asked about signs and symptoms of shijar, the answers were skin eruption (80 percent), body aches (62 percent), nasal voice and watery nasal discharge (34 percent). No one mentioned primary lesions on the external genitalia or lips.

Bodyaches are one of the most common and striking complaints in Turaba, especially among Bedouins. Taking the history of morbidity in the last two weeks of the study from 258 males and 325 females, 30 percent of the males (for all communities) said they had bodyaches. Twenty-one percent of the settled females and 50 percent of Bedouin females (a statistically significant difference) complained of bodyaches. From the records of the outpatients of the local health center, more than 20 percent of all complaints were from bodyaches.

In general the people in Turaba believe in two main causes of disease; supernatural power, and physical agents with no specific knowledge about pathogenesis. However, they are more knowledgeable about shijar. Eighty-five heads of households were asked about the possible cause of transmission of Shijar. Most of the answers were that it occured because of sexual contact and using the same utensils for drinking and eating. Other answers were "from God," "from mother to child through breast milk," or "if one drank from any utensil contaminated by a dog."

Traditionally, Shijar is treated by drinking hot wolf meat soup. Pepper and plenty of animal fat are added to it and the patient is then heavily covered so that he sweats a great deal and the disease is expelled from his body. It is interesting to compare this folk medicine treatment with the medieval medicine fever therapy for syphilis, which was in vogue up until the 1950s.

VDRL Test:

The agreement between FTA and VDRL test is shown in Table 2.

Table 2. Correlation Between FTA and VDRL Tests.

	FTA		
	+	−−	**Total**
VDRL +	7	−−	7
−−	11	64	75
Total	18	64	82

Co-positivity = 39 percent, Co-negativity = 100 percent, Overall agreement =85 percent.

Buck[7] in his study of Ethopia compared the two tests and found a higher co-positively (69 percent), and a lower co-negatively (77 percent) with a less overall agreement (74.6 percent).

Discussion

Respondents of different age groups (except 0-5 years in the settled community) showed reactions to the FTA test ranging from 6 percent in the settled community to 25 percent in the Bedouin community. This might indicate either venereal syphilis or endemic syphilis (Bejel). In favor of venereal syphilis was the observance of a few cases of gonorrhea in the main town. The polygamy practice, although limited, the frequency of divorce and remarriage, and the migration of young men to the cities for work may account for this.

The evidence for endemic syphilis is, however, more striking. The moral code among Bedouins is very high. They are very strict about premarital and extramarital sexual contacts. In the latter case death is the normal penalty.

Most of the literature refers to endemic syphilis (Bejel) as a non-venereal disease prevalent in Bedouin communities. One probable method of transmission is the use of common eating and drinking utensils. Use of common utensils is normal practice in Turaba. Overcrowding and poor sanitary conditions are other factors in spreading the disease.

At the time of the survey we were surprised by the high percentage of complaints of bodyache from outpatients. Among the possible reasons for increased prevalence of bodyaches are the inadequate insulation in tents against the great changes in temperature, possible salt depletion cramps due to high summer temperatures, Vitamin D deficiency particularly in females, and the high prevalence of arthritis and rheumatism. The common complaint of bodyaches could possibly be caused by the high prevalence of Shijar. The question needs further investigation.

Summary and Conclusion

Most of the available literature on the subject refers to endemic syphilis as a disease of Bedouins and semi-Bedouins. Some refer to Saudi Arabia as an island of endemic syphilis.

By examining the sera of 107 participants, both settled and Bedouin, in Turaba the FTA test revealed positive results in up to 25 percent of the 15 to 19 percent years age group among Bedouins. Examining the sera of nine Bedouin patients who attended the health center complaining of Shijar, seven were positively reactive to the FTA test. Up to 50 percent of the women in the Bedouin community complained of bodyaches in the last two weeks of the study, and from the records of the health center, bodyache is the most prevalent complaint. This might be due to Shijar since there appears to be no other explanation.

Considering the high moral code against extramarital sexual contact of the Turaba Bedouin, the low sanitary conditions, the usual habit of drinking from a common utensil, the absence of congenital syphilis or suggestive history of syphilis among mothers under the study, we can assume that much of the disease is endemic and not venereal syphilis.

We conclude that endemic syphilis is prevalent in Saudi Arabia. The problem deserves action in terms of epidemiological surveys and organized control.

Follow up Comments

Two studies have been conducted in the late 1970s to explore the magnitude of treponemal infections in Saudi Arabia. The first study was conducted by Pace[8] who investigated clinically and serologically 2515 individuals attending Tabuk military hospital in the period between 1976-80. Following is an excerpt of his findings.

- Non-venereal endemic syphilis exists in considerable numbers among the nomadic communities (up to 17 percent of the investigated cases were serologically positive). Venereal syphilis is much less common and almost exclusively limited to urban population.

- Endemic syphilis has become clinically attenuated within the last 30 years, possibly because of the improved hygienic conditions among nomads.

- At least 5 percent of the population in certain endemic areas have the active disease.

The author debated the possible impact of improving socioeconomic conditions versus massive treatment. His conclusion was that intelligent use of penicillin can speed up the process of control or even eradication.

The second study was conducted by Chowdhury et al[9] among 1572 attendants of the outpatient clinic at King Abdul Aziz Hospital in Riyadh between 1978 - 1980. Serologically 6.6 percent of the cases were positive.

Most of the cases were Saudi males aged 20 to 29 years. The authors suggested that with the exception of one or two cases the disease was venereally transmitted.

The findings of these two studies do not reflect the situation of treponemiasis in Saudi Arabia since they were carried out in hospitals. The sample in the first study was predominantly from Bedouin population and it showed endemic syphilis as the main problem, whereas the second study was carried out mainly among city dwellers and showed venereal syphilis as the main problem.

Apparently there is a great need for immediate action to study the epidemiology of treponemiasis (venereal and non-venereal) in Saudi Arabia and to implement a control program.

BIBLIOGRAPHY

1. Grin El. Endemic Syphilis in Bosnia. Bulletin World Health Organization 1952; 7:1 - 74.

2. Guthe TC. Die Bekampfung de Endimishen Syphilis in Entwicklungslandern. Archiv fur Klinishe und Experimentalle Dermatologic Gesellshaft, Band 1964; 219: 194-210.

3. Franklin HT. Communicable and Infectious Diseases; Diagnosis, Prevention and Treatment. St. Louis: The C.V. Mosby Company, 1964: 691-702.

4. Hudson EH. Treponematosis in Perspective. Bulletin World Health Organization 1965; 32: 735-748.

5. Ghouroury AA. The Syphilis Problem in Asir Province, Saudi Arabia. Bulletin World Health Organization 1954; 10: 691-702.

6. Luger Anton. Non-venereally Transmitted Endemic Syphilis in Vienna. British Journal of Venereal Disease 1972; 48: 356.

7. Buck AA, Spruyt DJ. Seroreactivity in the Venereal Disease Research Laboratory Slide Tests and the Fluorescent Treponemal Antibody Test. American Journal of Hygiene, July 1964; Vol. 80; 1: 91-102.

8. Pace JL. Treponematoses in Arabia/Endemic Nonvenereal Syphilis (Begel) in Saudi Arabia. Saudi Medical Journal 1983; 4:211-217

9. Chowdhury MNH et al. Incidence of Treponimal Infection in Different Clinics at King Abdul Aziz Teaching Hospital, Riyadh, Saudi Arabia. Saudi Medical Journal 1982; 3.1: 31-34.

Cholera Epidemic In Jizan District

In July 1972, an epidemic of cholera broke out in Jizan distict (estimated population 655,000) in the southwestern part of Saudi Arabia, on the northern borders of Yemen. In the beginning there were several cases of uninvestigated diarrhea in different localities in Jizan district. The first reported case of cholera was a 35-year-old Yemeni male who had arrived from Yemen to visit relatives a few days prior to becoming ill. Within a few days of his arrival several cases of diarrhea and vomiting appeared among his relatives and neighbors. From swabs of the victims, and water samples from household utensils and the village water holes, vibrio cholera, biotype El-Tor, serotype Inaba was repeatedly isolated. A campaign was promptly started to control the epidemic in the district and manpower, equipment, supplies and vehicles were mobilized.

The district (Figure 7, page 32) is divided into three areas, Jizan City, Samta and Sabia. Two general hospitals in Jizan City and Sabia and a secondary school in Samta were converted into isolation hospitals. The headquarters of the campaign was in Jizan city and teams of doctors, nurses, medical orderlies, assistant sanitarians and home visitors were stationed in each of the three hospitals. The main emphasis was given to:

1. Cordon sanitair around Jizan district.

2. Strict surveillance of all reported cases and contacts.

3. Mass vaccination.

4. Mass prophylaxis with antibacterial drugs.

5. Environmental sanitation and water chlorination.

Primary vaccination using El-Tor vibrio vaccine, 1 cc intramuscular for adults and 0.5 cc for children, was started in the villages where the cases were reported and extended to the surrounding villages.

At the same time, chemoprophylactic agent (Terramycin then Chloromycetin) was given to every vaccinated person (1 gm daily for three days for adults, half dose for children).

Surveillance, water sampling, water chlorination and sanitary measures were carried on at the same time.

The epidemic was brough under control in six weeks. In all, 286 cases were admitted to the three hospitals in the whole Jizan district. This paper deals with some epidemiological features of the 109 cholera patients who were admitted to Jizan city hospital.

Results

The distribution of the 109 cholera patients by age, sex and nationality is shown in Table 3.

From Table 3, we find that 55 percent of patients were Saudi and 45 percent were Yemeni and that 47 percent were males and 53 percent females. The highest percentage of cases was among children under 10 years of age. If this reflects the picture of the community, it could indicate endemicity of the disease.[1] There is, however, no reliable statistical data on age, sex and nationality distribution of the population resident in Jizan district.

In addition to diarrhea and vomiting, dehydration was experienced by 74 percent of the patients. The age groups, up-to-nine years and the over-fifty years old, experienced a higher percentage of dehydration than average (80 percent and 82 percent respectively. Table 4).

Out of the total 109 patients, 15 had received cholera vaccine, as well as chemoprophylaxis during two weeks before admission, whereas of the 94 patients who did not receive vaccine or chemoprophylaxis, 69 (73 percent) were dehydrated at the time of admission (Table 5). Every patient was treated for dehydration with Ringer-lactate solution and antibiotic therapy with tetracyclin.

Five out of 109 hospitalized patients died, all of them suffering from severe diarrhea and dehydration. Three were children below nine years of age and two were adults over 40 years old, all of them came from villages some distance from the hospital. Only one had received cholera vaccine and chemoprophylaxis 10 days before admission.

Discussion

No reliable data is available on the number of Yemeni residents in Jizan district, however, many of them live in Jizan in groups, or pass through it on their way to other cities in Saudi Arabia, looking for work or performing the pilgrimage during the season.

The WHO weekly epidemiological record of March 10, 1972 declared Yemen as a cholera-infected area while Saudi Arabia had been cholera-free for the previous two years. The last epidemic was in 1970 in the eastern region of the country and was due to Ogawa strain.

The first reported case of cholera in the present epidemic was a Yemeni male visiting his relatives in Jizan. Of the cholera patients admitted to Jizan hospital, 45 percent were Yemenis. These facts suggest that cholera was imported from Yemen across the borders of southwest Saudi Arabia.

The high prevalence of dehydration among patients (74 percent) could be explained by the wide distribution of the small villages in Jizan district, long distance and rough roads. Although more than 30 vehicles were used in the campaign as well as a helicopter for rapid transportation of staff and supplies and for ferrying patients from remote areas to the hospital, many patients arrived in an advanced condition.

The reluctance of the people of Jizan to report immediately their sick, either in the hope that they would be cured by God, with the help of native medicine, or to avoid the nuisance of home visits or rectal swabs, intensified these problems. For the same reasons there was incomplete coverage of chemoprophylaxis and vaccination for the population concerned.

Many of the patients admitted came from areas not yet covered by immunization and chemoprophylaxis. Only 15 out of the total 109 patients had a history of cholera innoculations and chemoprophylaxis. However, no statistically significant differences were found in the symptoms (dehydration) or prognosis (death) between those who had vaccine and chemoprophylaxis, and those who had not.

For the first two weeks of the campaign, terramycin was given as chemoprophylaxis and chemotherapy. Then the central laboratory in Riyadh showed that chloromycetin was more effective and accordingly chemoprophylaxis and treatment were changed to chloromycetin. Cluff has stated that terramycin is the drug of choice in the treatment of cholera, with a hastening of the disappearance of vibrio cholera from the feces.[2] The WHO Expert Committee on Cholera reported that terramycin and chloromycetin are equally effective.[3]

From field trials[4,5] we know that vaccination and chemoprophylaxis lower the incidence of morbidity but does not change the clinical picture once the organisms have created their toxins.

Conclusion

The epidemic of cholera which broke out in 1972 in Jizan district in southwest Saudi Arabia was probably imported from Yemen.

Cultural barriers resulted in delaying reporting of patients and consequently late admission with a high percentage of dehydration.

There was no apparent difference in morbidity between those who received cholera vaccine and chemoprophylaxis and those who did not receive them. The sample size was relatively small, but the results indicate the need of further field work on the effect of immunization and chemoprophylaxis on prognosis.

Table 3. Distribution of Cholera Patients by Age, Sex and Nationality.

Age (years)	Sex			Nationality		
	Male	Female	Total	Saudi	Yemeni	Total
0 - 9	16	14	30	18	12	30
10 - 19	10	8	18	13	5	18
20 - 29	6	10	16	8	8	16
30 - 39	9	10	19	9	10	19
40 - 49	6	9	15	7	8	15
50+	4	7	11	5	6	11
Total	51	58	109	60	49	109

Table 4. Distribution of Choler? Patients by Age and Presence of Dehydration-

Age	Dehydrated		Non-dehydrated		Total	
	No.	%	No.	%	No.	%
0 9	24	80	6	20	30	100
10 - 19	12	67	6	33	18	100
20 - 29	12	75	4	25	16	100
30 - 39	14	74	5	26	19	100
40 - 49	10	67	5	33	15	100
50+	9	82	2	18	11	100

Table 5. Realtion Between Presence of Dehydration and Reception of Vaccine and Chemoprophlaxis.

Cases	Received	Vaccine Not Received	Total
Dehydrated	12	69	81
Non-dehydrated	3	25	28
Total	15	94	109

BIBLIOGRAPHY

1. World Health Organization. Principles and Practice of Cholera Control. WHO 1970, Public Health Paper; 40: 25.

2. Gluff LE. Cecil-Loeb Textbook of Medicine. 13th ed. Philadelphia: Saunders Co., 1971: 590.

3. WHO Expert Committee on Cholera. WHO Technical Report Series, 1959: 179.

4. Oseasohn RO, Benson AS. Field Trial of Cholera Vaccine in East Pakistan. Lancet 1955; 1: 449-50.

5. WHO. A Controlled Field Trial of Effectiveness of Cholera El-Tor Vaccines in the Philippines. Bulletin of World Health Organizaton. 1970; 38: 917-23.

Cutaneous Leishmaniasis in Bisha

Bisha district is a wide area about 40,000 square kilometers, situated in the southwest of Saudi Arabia (Figure 17, p. 152) and has a population of approximately 104,000. The inhabitants live in more than 400 small villages, oases and settlement areas of Bedouins, widely scattered along six valleys. Twenty percent of the population are still nomads.

Bisha town (pop. 20,000), the capital of Bisha district, is surrounded by small villages, settlement areas and nomadic sub-tribes. There is a central hospital in Bisha and 23 health centers, providing primary health care, throughout the area.

During the summer of 1974, a few cases of cutaneous leishmaniasis were seen in the outpatient clinic of Bisha hospital. An increasing number of cases were reported by various health centers. Before that time the disease was almost unknown in Bisha.

Materials and Methods

This study was conducted in October 1974 in Bisha hospital. Among 620 patients who attended the dermatology outpatient clinic during that month, 110 cases of cutaneous leishmaniasis were identified. Of these 73 came from Bisha town, 28 from four small villages within five kilometers of Bisha and the remaining nine came from remote villages. All except six were Saudi.

The patients were clinically examined and two smear slides taken from each. After removal of the covering scales, a bunch of tissue was taken from the indurated edge; smears were fixed in methyl alcohol and stained with Giemsa (one drop to one ml.). Only 103 patients were examined; seven refused to give smears. Patients were treated with Sodium Stibogluconate B.P. (Pentostam) for the first time in Saudi Arabia.

Results

Five patients were less than one year old. The highest incidence was among the 58 patients in the one to 10 year age group. The incidence of the infection became increasingly less common in the higher age groups. The lowest incidence was among the age group 31 years and over, in which there were 13 patients. Both sexes were similarly affected (Table 6).

Various types of lesions were seen. Ninety percent were of the classical dry type but verrucous and acuminated types were also seen. Most of the lesions were less than two cm. in diameter.

In 88 patients a single lesion was the predominant feature; in 21 patients the number ranged from two to five. In one patient, however, 16 lesions were counted. Infection occurred on the exposed parts of the body. The most common site was the face (Table 7).

Of the 103 cases examined, 73 showed Leishmania bodies in smears. In lesions with secondary infection, smears were frequently negative and Leishmania could only be demonstrated after cleaning the ulcers and reexamining them on alternative days. Only four patients had scars from old lesions together with active ones.

Before the survey Fouadin and Resochin were applied for treatment without much success. We tried, for the first time in Saudi Arabia, Sodium Stibogluconate B.P. (Pentostam) for treatment of patients under the survey.

Sodium Stibogluconate B.P. (kindly supplied by Burroughs and Wellcome Co., England) in sterile stable solution containing the equivalent of 100 gm. of pentavalent antimony per ml. was used parenterally. Infants less than one year and those in the one to five year age group were given one and 1.5 ml. intramuscularly as an initial dose and subsequent daily dose of two and three ml. respectively. Age group six to 11 years and 12 and over were given IV as an initial dose two and three ml. and subsequent daily dose of four and six ml. respectively. Patients were kept under observation for an hour after the injection. After completion of the last dose, patients were followed-up for two weeks to evaluate the results.

The clinical response as shown by healing of the lesions was confirmed in most cases by the inability to find leismania bodies in smears from pre-treatment positive ones. The drug was not given to patients with liver, kidney, heart or debilitating disease, or to pregnant women.

Only 56 patients continued receiving the treatment daily for six to 15 days. Fifty four refused treatment or failed to continue and thus are not reported. The results are shown in Table 8.

Good result: moderate softening of the granulation base and diminution of the size; no parasite but no cicitrization.

Excellent result: marked dimunation of the size, no parasite in smears and beginning of cicatrization.

Table 6. Age and Sex of Leishmania patients.

Age Group	Male	Female	Total	Positive Smear
1 — 10	29	29	58	44
11 — 20	11	12	23	15
21 — 30	9	7	16	9
31 +	8	5	13	5
Total	57	53	110	73

Table 7. Distribution of Leishhmania Lesions.

Site	Single Lesions	Multiple Lesions
Face	24	
Nose	13	
Ear	1	various
Neck	1	
Upper limbs	25	sites
Lower limbs	23	
Other sites	1	
Number of Patients	88	22

Table 8. Prognosis Related to Number of Injections in Different Age Groups.

No. of Injections	No. of cases	Results Obtained		
		Poor	Good	Excellent
6 - 7	10	10	--	--
8 - 10	40	2	21	17
11 - 15	6	--	2	4
Total	56	12	23	21

Mild side effects such as pruritic skin eruption, anorexia, general aches and fatigue were observed in six patients; five of them continued the course with symptomatic treatment and one was discontinued.

Discussion

Most people do not have any name for the disease. However, a few call it Al Mohtafera (the digger) or Al Moktawiya (treated by cautery). In Riyadh it is called Okht, Nafra or Al Dommal.[1] The native treatment is to burn a piece of dried camel skin and cauterize the lesion. Such destructive methods of treatment, used for a long time in modern medicine and involving the application of caustic substances such as sulphuric acid and potassium permanganate, always raised controversial issues.

The incidence is high among children, an indication of the existence of endemic foci in the area.

The number of lesions varies greatly. In the present study, up to 16 were counted. In other studies, 75 were reported in Riyadh[2] and 123 in Iraq.[3] Multiple lesions could be explained by simultaneous infection or by recent sandfly bites.[4]

The results in patients treated with Pentostam varied from poor (12), to good (23), to excellent (21). A better response was met in: (a) patients of a young age group (less than 2 years); (b) lesions on the face, ears and hands (sun exposed); (c) lesions with short durations and, (d) patients receiving 11 to 15 injections. Also, accuminated and verroucous types of lesions gave less satisfactory results than the classical ones. Two infected cases responded well after treatment with antibiotics.

Manson-Bahr, in 1959[5], obtained good results with the drug against resistant cases of East African Kala Azar. Abdella et al.[6] in 1973 reported that in Sudan cutaneous leishmaniasis responds well to the drug. In the present study, pentostam gave satisfactory results.

Conclusion

A proper survey of natural leishmaniasis foci in Saudi Arabia is needed to clarify the factors controlling the spread of infection in the human population. Epidemiological investigations into the vector, reservoir host and the human disease are important for working out an effective system of leishmaniasis control. Investigation on better methods of early diagnosis and treatment should continue.

Follow-up Comments

The reports from the Ministry of Health show an increasing number of cutaneous leismaniasis cases from 1395 H. to 1401 H. (1975-1981) (Table 9).

People in many localities experienced the disease for the first time in their lives. The theory behind the new waves of the epidemic is the expansion of small towns and villages which brought inhabitants into closer contact with the reservoir hosts, gerbals and rodents. This is an obscure area which needs applied research in epidemiology and control.

Table 9. Number of Cases of Cutaneous Leishmaniasis Reported by the Ministry; of Health 1395 - 1401 AH. (1975 - 1981 AD).

Year	No of Reported Cases
1395	7
1396	52
1397	119
1398	1043
1399	2469
1400	3471
1401	3302

BIBLIOGRAPHY

1. Morsey TA, Shoura MI. Treatment of Saudi Arabian Cutaneous Leishmaniasis, Journal of Tropical Medicine and Hygiene 1974; 77: 68.

2. Morsey TA, Shoura MI. Natural Leishmania Infection Sought in Animals in El Kharj, Saudi Arabi. Journal of the Egyptian Public Health Association 1975; 50: 328.

3. Rahim GF, Tatar IH. Oriental Sore in Iraq. Bulletin Endemic Disease 1966; 8: 29.

4. Moskovskij SD, Southgate BA. Clinical Aspects of Leishmaniasis with Special Reference to the USSR. Bulletin World Health Organization 1971; 44: 491.

5. Manson-Bahr PEC. Transactions of the Royal Society of Tropical Medicine and Hygiene 1959; 53: 123.

6. Abdella RE, Ali M, Wasfi Al, El-Hassan AM. Transaction of the Royal Society of Tropical Medicine and Hygiene 1973: 67: 549.

Filariasis in the Western Part of Saudi Arabia

Wuchereria bancrofti causes Bancroft's Filariasis, a very old and serious disease. The ancient Hindus (600 B.C.) diagnosed the disease and an Arab physician, Ibn-Sina (Avicenna) described its dramatic clinical picture. It was referred to as "elephantiasis arabicum." In 1866, Wucherer discovered in Brazil the presence of microfilariasis in chylous urine. Sir Patrick Manson in 1878[1] reported that Culex quinquefasciatus (Syn. C. fatigans) was an intermediate host and described the noctural activity of the microfilariasis in peripheral blood and diurnal concentration in the lung.

Bancroft's filariasis is indigenous in practically all the warm regions of the world, from about 41° north to about 28° south, although it is not evenly distributed or uniformly prevalent in any country. In 1947 Stoll[2] estimated the combined infection from Bancroft's and Malayan filariasis to be about 189 million, of which 157 million were in Asia. It is prevalent in Asia, the coasts of Arabia, Malaya, Formosa, China, the southern part of Korea, Japan and South Pacific Islands.[3] Also, Manson-Bahr in 1945[4] referred to southwestern Arabia as an infested area.

Twenty-three cases of filariasis bancrofti (serologically and parasitologically positive) were reported by the central laboratory in Riyadh in 1972. Fourteen of them were Yemeni immigrant workers, seven were Saudis and the remaining two were of other nationalities. Five out of seven Saudis were originally from the western part of the Kingdom and had no history of travel outside the country. During a recent malaria surveillance, Culex fatigans (vector of W. bancrofti) was reported in different areas including Makkah in the west and Jizan in the southwest.

No scientific studies have been made on filariasis in Saudi Arabia. The present study was carried out to throw light on the magnitude of the problem. The western area was chosen as a center for the study on the basis that a) five positive Saudi cases came from there, b) the presence of many immigrant Yemeni workers, c) the assumptions of Augustine[3] and Manson-Bahr,[4] and d) the presence of the vectors. In addition, Jeddah, Makkah and Taif are among the main centers for foreign pilgrims.

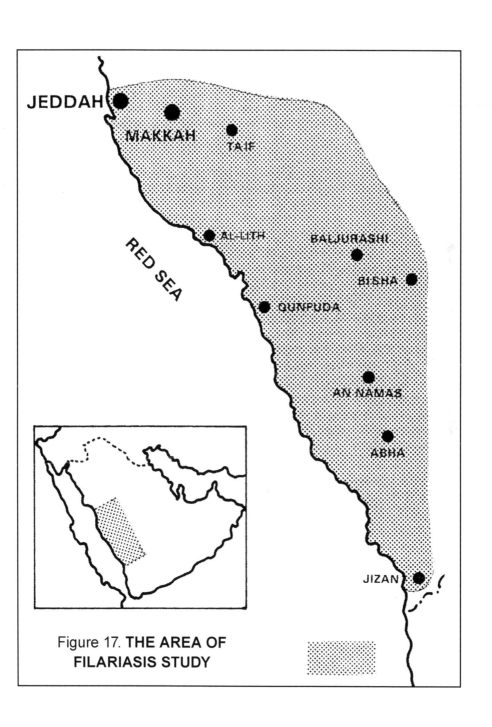

Figure 17. **THE AREA OF FILARIASIS STUDY**

Material and Method

Two field trips were arranged to the western region of the country (Figure 17). The first trip was for one month to the cities of Makkah, Jeddah and Taif and their environs during the 'Haj' season of 1394 A.H. (December 1973). At this time about two million Muslims from all over the world gather in this area for the pilgrimage. The aim was to explore the prevalence of the disease among samples of both Saudis and foreign pilgrims. The second trip was in 1974 for one month to the Asir highlands and the coastal area.

Studies were carried out to a) detect and identify the vector, and b) explore the presence of the human disease.

a. Mosquitoes, mainly Culex, were collected in great numbers by various methods using New Jersey mosquito light traps which were positioned near water beds, fields and vegetation. In addition, domestic mosquitoes were collected indoors by aspirators. Some of the collected specimens were preserved in labeled bottles of 70 percent alcohol. Others were put in small cardboard boxes filled with damp cotton wool. They were then sent to the central laboratory in Riyadh.

b. A team from the Malaria Division of the Ministry of Health was sent to the area under study to collect samples of peripheral blood. Groups of households were selected randomly in urban, semi-urban and rural communities. Thin and thick blood films were taken around midnight (10 p.m. to 2 a.m.) from all members of selected households. About 150 to 250 samples from each community were collected, making a total of 1,568 slides.

Thin films were fixed in absolute methly alcohol (acetone free) for one to two minutes. Thick films required no fixing since dehemoglobinization was necessary. Slides were then stained in Giemsa's stain (one drop to one ml.) for about 30 minutes, washed off and dried in air. Groups of hospitals, health centers, schools and markets were visited. Meetings and discussions were held with physicians, teachers, sheikhs and key informants. A few cases with clinical manifestations were spotted and examined.

Results

A. Vector:

The collection of insects yielded a variety of genera and species. Of interest are the following:

1. Culex pipiens complex
2. Culex fatigans
5. Aedes sp.
6. Theobaldia sp.*
7. Culicoides puncticollis*
*Not recorded before in this area.

3. Anopheles multicolor
4. Anopheles turkhudi
8. Culicoides riethi*
9. Phlebotomus sp.*
10. Some chironomids

B. Human Disease:

The clinical picture of the 23 cases of elephantiasis reported by the Central Public Health Laboratory, Riyadh, in 1972 is shown in Table 10.

Table 10. Clinical Findings of 23 Cases of Filariasis According to Sex and Nationality.

Clinical picture	Sex	No.	Nationality Saudi	Yemeni	Others
Enlargement of lower limb (uni-or bilateral)	M	8	1	6	1
	F	4	2	1	1
Enlargement of genitalia	M	7	3	4	---
	F	2	1	1	---
Enlargement of lower limb and genitalia	M	2	---	2	---
Total	M+F	23	7	14	2

All 23 cases gave a positive skin response to antigen prepared from Dirofilaria immitis in dilution 1:8,000 (supplied by WHO). On the other hand, microfilariasis were only recovered from six Yemenis by examination of the sediment from two ml. of blood mixed with 10 ml. of 2 percent formaldehyde, centrifuged for five minutes at 2,000 rpm.

Most of the physicians, teachers and sheikhs with whom we discussed the problem of elephantitis had never seen this condition in the areas visited. A few mentioned seeing sporadic cases.

During the first trip to the field two cases of filariasis (serologically and parasitologically positive) were detected in Makkah and Taif. The first was a 50-year-old Nigerian pilgrim with elephantitis of the right lower limb. The second was an 18-year-old Yemeni with two years residence in Makkah and a long history of elephantitis of the right lower limb and genitalia.

On the second trip (1974), three cases of elephantitis were detected. They were Saudi nationals with no history of travel outside the country.

The first case was a 22-year-old male with elephantitis of the right lower limb, enlarged right inguinal lymph nodes, and old scars in the right groin. He had contracted the disease when he was 10 years old living in the nomadic community of Thurba, 17 kilometers from Abha. He had experienced attacks of fever, bodyaches, vomiting, anorexia, dizziness and tenderness of the right lower limb almost every six months. The attacks lasted about 10 days. Enlargement of the right lower limb gradually increased. The attacks had recently become more frequent. He had been hospitalized four times without very much improvement. A blood survey was carried out in Thurba and Omara, the nearest village. All results were negative.

The second case was a 45-year-old Saudi male from the village of Makarma, two kilometers from Baljurashy, with severe elephantitis of the right lower limb. He contracted the disease at the age of 20 years when he was resident in Makkah. Blood surveys were carried out in Makarma and in the district where he had lived in Makkah. All midnight blood films were negative, and the patient himself was parasitologically negative.

The third case was a 32-year-old female from Sabt al Alaia in the Hejaz mountains. She had elephantitis of the vulva. It had started two years before as an abcess in the right inguinal region while whe was residing in her own village. Six months earlier she had been in Bisha and two years before that she lived in Riyadh. A blood film was negative.

Table 11 shows the number of persons examined for thin and thick blood films. The blood samples were collected at random (10 p.m. to 2 a.m.) during the second field trip (1974). The only positive slide was from a Yemeni in Leith. Three slides showed microfilariasis of Dipetalonema perstans (non-pathogenic till now). Sixteen slides were positive for Plasmodium falciparum.

Table 11. Number of Persons Examined for Thin and Thick Blood Films.

Area	Total No.	Saudi	Non-Saudi
Makkah	33	29	4
Taif	240	231	9
Thurba & Omara	207	194	13
Makarma	278	264	14
Bal-garn	60	52	8
Bisha	55	49	6
Leith	274	257	17
Qunfodah	201	187	14
Jizan	220	183	37
Total	1,568	1,446	122

Discussion

The foregoing data dealt with 28 cases (Saudis and non-Saudis) with clinical manifestations, 23 reported by the Public Health Laboratory in Riyadh and five detected during the field trips. Twenty-five cases were skin tested with a positive response. Only one showed microfilariae in peripheral blood while six showed microfilariae by the concentration method of Knott.[5]

Microfilariae are frequently absent especially in elephantitis cases. Chandler in 1960[6] suggested that clinical signs and symptoms must be relied on to a considerable extent.

Transmission of W. bancrofti, in contrast to malaria and yellow fever, is by no means limited to one genus or group of mosquitoes. Abut 60 species of mosquitoes including members of Culex, Anopheles, Aedes, Psorophora and Mansonia throughout the world serve as natural biological transmitters.[7] Of these, only a few species, all closely associated with man and which prefer his blood, are common transmitters. The following are particularly important.[8]

1. Culex quinquefasciatus (Syn = C. fatigans)

2. Culex pipiens and Culex p. var. pallens

3. Aedes aegypti

4. Aedes polynesiensis

5. Anopheles darlingi

6. Anopheles gambiae

7. Anopheles punctualatus var. farauti, molluccensis and punctualatus

In the western part of Saudi Arabia, the following species have been reported.

1. Culex pipiens complex

2. Culex fatigans

3. Aedes aegypti

4.   Anopheles gambiae (among 12 species of Anopheles in that area)

All of these have proved naturally good vectors for W. bancrofti in many countries such as China, India, West Africa, Egypt, Congo, Zanzibar and Brazil.

The existence of 10 Saudi cases, eight of which came from the western part of Saudi Arabia and with no history of movement outside the country, suggests the evidence of endemic foci in the area. The rapid process of urbanization and Bedouin settlement, and reported filaria vectors in different areas of the country, indicate the possibility of further spreading of the disease.

Human aggregation reduces the distance between houses or dwellings to within this limited flight range.[10]

Summary and Conclusion

Twenty-three cases of elephantiasis (seven Saudi and 16 non-Saudis), all of whom showed a positive skin response, were reported to the Central Public Health Laboratory in Riyadh in 1972. Five of the Saudi cases originally came from the western part of Saudi Arabia.

As a result, two surveys were carried out in different areas in Saudi Arabia to explore the prevalence and epidemiology of the disease. Four vectors were found, 1568 midnight blood films were examined and only one positive and another five cases of elephantiasis (three Saudis) were detected.

The conclusion was that filariasis does exist in small foci in western Saudi Arabia, with the possibility of spreading because of the favorable conditions created by the rapid process of urbanization and settlement as well as increasing contact with the outside world.

BIBLIOGRAPHY

1. Manson P. Chinese Customs Med Repts. 1878; 3: 1.

2. Stoll NR. Journal of Parasitology; 1947; 33: 1.

3. Augustine DL. New York State Journal of Medicine; 1945; 45: 495.

4. Manson-Bahr PH. In: Manson's Tropical Disease. 16th ed. London 1945.

5. Knott JI. Transactions of the Royal Society Tropical Medicine and Hygiene. 1939; 33: 191.

6. Chandler AC, Read CP. Introduction of Parasitology. 10th ed: U.S.A. 1960.

7. Lincicome DR. In: Craig and Faust. Clinical Parasitology. 6th ed. Philadelphia; 1957.

8. Faust EC, Russel PE. Clinical Parasitology. 7th ed. Philadelphia; 1964.

9. Lavoipierre MMJ. Annals of Tropical Medicine and Parasitology; 1958; 52: 326.

10. Crosskey RW. Annals of Tropical Medicine and Parasitology; 1954; 48: 152.

Leprosy and Leprosy Care

In this study, selected clinico-epidemiological features of the 144 inpatients in Hadda Leprosy Hospital are discussed. In addition, the knowledge and attitude of a sample of 220 people towards leprosy is examined. The results are intended to be used as a base line for an epidemiological survey of leprosy in Saudi Arabia where little is known about the disease.

The leprosy Hospital in Hadda, 35 kilometers from Jeddah, is the only leprosy hospital in Saudi Arabia. It has 180 beds and 144 patients. The cases are usually referred informally to the hospital from general hospitals, health centers and private clinics throughout the country. No other hospital in Saudi Arabia admits leprous patients.

The patients in Hadda Hospital are under the care of three physicians, eight nurses and a social worker. Records are incomplete and laboratory services inadequate. Moreover, there is no physiotherapy or rehabilitation program.

Methodology

The study was conducted in 1977, all 144 patients were examined clinically and their medical and social histories were recorded. Nasal scrapings from all 144 patients were obtained and transferred to Riyadh to be examined for M. leprae in the Central Laboratory. Biopsies were taken from only 11 cases due to patient resistance.

A questionnaire on the knowledge of cause of the disease, means of spread, and methods of protection, was directed to a random sample of 220 people (118 males and 102 females), residents of al Monfoh district, Riyadh city, who have moved in recently from various parts of the Kingdom. They are all adults, mostly with basic elementary education.

Results

The Hadda Hospital Patients

Of the total 144 patients, 64 had tuberculoid leprosy, 69 lepromatus leprosy and 11 borderline lesions. The nasal scrapings from 119 were negative for M. leprae. This test is, however, affected by treatment and is of low sensitivity.

Ten patients were under 20 years of age and the ratio of males to females was 5:1 (Table 12); 72 of the patients were Saudi, 63 Yemeni and nine were other nationalities (Table 13).

Of the total 144 patients, 116 were illiterate. Of the 120 male patients, 71 were farmers, 12 laborers, seven nomadic Bedouins and the remainder had a variety of occupations. Patients in general were found to be of low socioeconomic class. No statistically significant difference was found between the three types of lesion in relation to nationality, education or occupation.

These findings are from an unrepresentative sample. In general health services are more accessible to adult males than to women and children Table 14 and Figure 18 show the areas of residence of the Saudi patients. Seventy percent of them are from the southwestern region of the country (containing 8 percent of the total area and 20 percent of the total population). This could indicate higher prevalence of the disease in that region.

Leprosy is known to be endemic in Yemen. The large number of Yemen laborers living in the southwestern region could influence the prevalence of the disease in this part of the Kingdom.

Laviron (unpublished observations) in his report on the Hadda Leprosy Hospital, obtained rather similar data. According to his report 69 percent of the patients were Saudi and the majority of the others were from Yemen. Of the Saudis, 39 percent were from the southwest.

Many factors, such as the size of the population, the social system, the health attitude and practice, and transportation facilities should be considered in interpreting this geographical distribution. Ninety-one patients (63 percent) were referred to the hospital without having had any specific care, whereas 15 (10 percent) mentioned that they had been treated by native practitioners. Of the 72 Saudi patients, 32 were complaining at their first contact with the hospital of irreversible deformities, such as claw hand, drop foot, mask-like face and lost fingers or toes. This is an indication of the late diagnosis and inefficient referral system.

A three-month supply of medicine is usually given to the patient on discharge. During the last three years, 297 discharged patients (250 males and 47 females) visited the outpatient department, with an average of two visits per patient. As there is no other center for leprosy care, this indicates an insufficient outpatient care and lack of community follow-up.

Table 12. Type of Leprosy According to Age and Sex.

Males: age (Years)	Borderline	Tuberculoid	Lepromatous	Total
		Type of leprosy		
--20	1	4	4	9
--30	5	22	14	41
--40	4	7	15	26
--50	--	9	7	16
50+	1	12	15	28
Total Males	11	54	55	120
Female: ages (Years)				
--20	--	--	1	1
--30	--	2	2	4
--40	--	1	5	6
--50	--	3	3	6
50+	--	4	3	7
Total Females	--	10	14	24
GRAND TOTAL	11	64	69	144

Table 13. Type of Leprosy According to Nationality.

Nationality:	Borderline	Type of leprosy Tuberculoid	Lepromatous	Total
Saudi	1	33	38	72
Yemeni	8	29	26	63
Others	2	2	5	9
Total	11	64	69	144

Forty-one patients had been in the hospital for more than four years. Some have been discharged and readmitted. Lepromatous lesions were found in 23 patients, borderline lesions in 14 and four had tuberculoid lesions.

The reasons for this lengthy stay or readmission are medical (five cases), social (11 cases) and a combination of both (24 cases). The main social reasons mentioned are "afraid of the hostile attitude of my neighbors," "nobody came to take me home," "I don't want to be a burden to my family" and "unable to work and earn my living."

Case Histories

CASE 1. Abdulla S., 55 years old, had tuberculoid leprosy with minimum disfiguration. He was discharged five years ago after being confirmed stationary. Life was difficult for him in his village so he came back to the hospital seeking readmission.

CASE 2. Fatima H. is in her 30s. She was admitted to the hospital three years ago. Her husband divorced her and her family refused to take her out of the hospital after the course of her treatment was completed. She is still in the hospital.

Table 14. Place of Residence of 72 Saudf Leprous Patients.

Region	Place of Residence	No. of Patients
Southwest	Jizan	25
	Asir	12
	Ghamid, Zahran	9
	Qunfuda	2
	Leith	1
West	Taif	7
	Jeddah	6
	Makkah	5
	Madinah	1
North	Qasim	1
East	Qatif	2
Central	Riyadh	1
Total		72

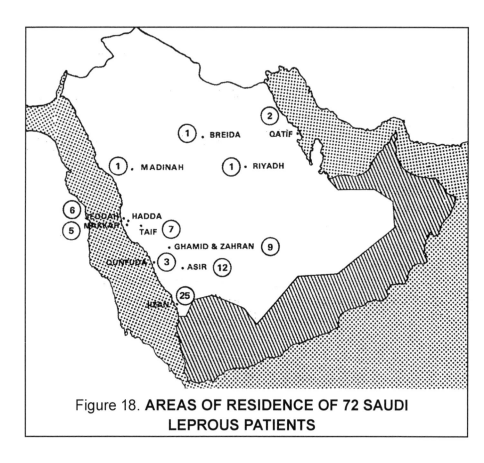

Figure 18. **AREAS OF RESIDENCE OF 72 SAUDI LEPROUS PATIENTS**

The patients in general suffer from the dilemma that the conditions in the hospital are not conducive to a prolonged stay and the outside world is not friendly.

Twenty-eight Saudis mentioned that they had prior contact with people suffering from leprosy, mostly members of their own families. A comprehensive list has been made of the contacts and their areas of residence for further epidemiological studies.

Knowledge and Attitude of the Public Towards the Disease.

Informal discussions on the subject of leprosy, 'Juzam' were held with several informed people of both sexes within various socioeconomic settings, including elderly people, sheiks and schoolmasters. A questionnaire was also completed with a sample of 220 residents of Al Manfoh district, Riyadh. The disease is considered highly contagious and is probably more feared than any other disease. Otherwise little is known about its causation, its manner of spreading and how individuals can be protected from it (Table 15). The questions were directed to the respondents as open-ended without specifying the answers, hence the non-specific responses.

Table 15. Answers of 220 Respondents to Questions on Leprosy.

Causes		Way of spread		Way of protection	
Don't know	126	Don't know	135	Don't know	136
From God	32	Personal Contact	61	Keep away From sick	54
Wearing wet clothes	14	Not contagious	5		
Bacteria	14	From God	2		
Dirt	10				

The question "If you have a son or daughter, would you let him/her marry a leprous patient?" was put to 116 of the respondents. One hundred and eight said "No." Among the reasons given were fear of infection and the deformity of a leper. Some of the informants believed native medicine to be the best remedy for the ailment.

"Take Al Oshba (some herbs grown in the desert), grind it, powder it and divide it into 40 small portions. Over 40 successive days the patient should boil a portion a day, inhale the steam and drink the extraction. Throughout the period he should be in isolation, away from the sunlight and he will be cured Inshallah, if God wills..."

Discussion

The striking feature is that patients tend to escape from life to the hospital, which in turn has the minimum comfort. They suffer from community rejection. This is indicated not only by the examples of Fatima and Abdulla, but also by the fact that 81 percent of the hospital patients are either single or divorced in a country where people, especially rural, marry early in life. The relatively high proportion of hospital patients of lepromatuous type may be due to the fact that such patients take refuge in the hospital.

The data from the hospital indicate late diagnosis, insufficient referral system, unnecessary length of stay in the hospital and inadequate hospital services in terms of diagnostic procedures and rehabilitation programs.

The public is ill-informed about the causation and the possibilities of treatment and prevention of the disease. Native medicine is still being practiced, probably more than is being admitted by the patients. This should not be ignored but rather evaluated and ameliorated. Native practitioners, who enjoy a great deal of esteem and respect, could be motivated to help in the campaign against the disease.

The lack of appropriate knowledge among the public results in a harsh and unsympathetic attitudes towards the sick, which consequently leads to emotional trauma, superimposed upon the physical handicap and disfiguration.

This is not unique to the present times, or to Saudi Arabia either. In medieval times the disease was considered "the great blight that threw its shadow over the daily life of medieval humanity. Fear of all other diseases together can hardly be compared to the terror caused by leprosy. A leper was treated inhumanely."

The Arabs feared the disease more than any other ailment. When Hareth Ibn Hilza-al-Yaskhuri (A.D. 550), suffering from leprosy (Wadah), was to recite his "Muallaka" before Amr Ibn-Hind, King of Al-Hira, Amr ordered a screen to be placed between them.

As a general impression and from the records of the Ministry of Health, leprosy does not appear to be a problem of a high magnitude in Saudi Arabia. From this study leprosy appears to exist in various parts of the Kingdom, especially in the southwestern region. The region in general is more over-populated than any other area in the Kingdom, economically less developed and has less health services. The geographical location of the region, adjacent to the Red Sea, close to sub-tropical and tropical Africa (where leprosy is endemic), could have affected the prevalence of the disease in this part of the Kingdom.

All data mentioned in this study should be considered with an understanding that the samples, both from the hospital and the community, are not representative of the country.

Characteristically, the patients are adult males, farmers, illiterate and of low socioeconomic status. This could reflect the attributes of leprous patients in the country, or that patients with different attributes are not represented because of lack of accessibility or social inhibitions.

Conclusion

The patients of Hadda Leprosy Hospital appear to make up only a fraction of the total number suffering from this disease in Saudi Arabia. Out of the 144 inpatients in Hadda Hospital, 72 are Saudi and 63 are Yemeni. Seventy percent of the Saudis came from the southwestern region and this would indicate that the disease is more prevalent there than elsewhere in Saudi Arabia.

Many of the patients come in at a late stage of the disease and may stay in hospital up to several years. Apparently, they face a stressful life in the community and take refuge in the hospital.

There is no active program for leprosy control in Saudi Arabia. Hadda Leprosy Hospital lacks many vital amenities and is located far from the southwestern region where the disease appears to have its highest incidence. As a result, both patients and their relatives face cultural and transportation problems.

The public is ill-informed about the disease, its causation, contagiousness and the possibilities of treatment and prevention. This, besides being a very fearful disease, leads to a harsh and unsympathetic attitude toward the sick.

We recommend the following: The integration of leprosy care in the primary health care system with emphasis on early detection, ambulatory care and rehabilitation programs, and the building of a new hospital in the southwest.

The use of the term "Hansen's disease" instead of leprosy may help in improving the attitude of the people towards the disease and its victims.

Follow-up Comments (1984)

The Leprosy Hospital was visited again in early 1984. Considerable progress has been noticed in the patients care compared to the situation in 1977. The pressing need to improve the unsatisfactory features of the hospital was given high priority by the authorities. A young, active and enthusiastic Saudi pharmacist had been appointed recently as director of the hospital and was given wide authority and financial support. He and his staff brought about a good deal of improvement. It is an indicative example of how effective decentralization of the health services system could be. Table 16 shows some of the changes achieved over the last eight years in the hospital.

Table 16. Some Changes in the Leprosy Hospital 1977 - 1984.

	1977	1984
Number of beds	180	200
Number of doctors	3	13
Number of nurses	8	50
Number of social workers	1	3
Number of other paramedicals	2	9
Inpatients: Total number	144	152

Percent of Saudi	72%	65%
Males to females	5-1	33-1
History of stay of four years or more	28%	38%
From West and Southwest Regions	70%	57%

The name of the hospital was changed from Leprosy Hospital to Ibn Sina Hospital which appears sensible. From the first instant the visitor can observe order, cleanliness and renovation of the old shabby and dirty building. New wings were added to accommodate the pharmacy, the laboratory and the dental clinics. The number of beds and number of patients have slightly increased but the quality of care, hygiene, recreation and nutrition are much better than before. Patients' record are impressive as well. The number of patients is too small to detect any significant differences in attributes. However, the increase of female to male ratio could mean better accessibility of hospital care to the female population.

The decrease in the percentage of the patients coming from the Southwest Region could be due to an improvement of the health situation in the Southwest Region, the rapid movement and resettlement of Saudi population, or a combination of factors. There is no significant change of the Saudi to non-Saudi ratio. The outpatients records show a new phenomenon. Over the three years 1974 to 1976 only 297 ambulatory patients were treated at the outpatient clinic. In contrast, in the year 1983, 762 patients were treated at the outpatient clinic. This is in addition to 1122 non-leprosy patients who attended the dermatology clinic. This could indicate better awareness of leprous patients of the need for ambulatory care, or a positive response by patients to the availability of better health services. A negative phenomenon was also observed. Out of 152 inpatients, 60 (49 males and 11 females) have a history of staying in the hospital for four years or more (38 percent of the total number), which is more than the percentage in 1977. Could it be the improvement in the hospital environment which encouraged the patients to extend their stay in the hospital, or rather the harsh and unfriendly attitude of the public towards the lepers that became even worse? The reader must be reminded that the hospital cannot discharge a patient against his or her will or if his or her relatives did not request the discharge, even if he or she is bacteriologically negative.

The hospital situation with all its improvements is still far from perfect. There is a need for a physiotherapy department, more recreational facilities, additional staff, especially Saudi (all physicians and nurses are non-Saudis).

Another missing aspect is the community-based activities such as surveillance, health education of the public, early detection of cases and rehabilitation programs. The hospital can be a recognized training center for medical students and health professionals. This would bring more resources to the hospital and upgrade its status.

RECOMMENDED LITERATURE

Arnold HL, Fasal P. Leprosy, Diagnosis and Management. Springfield Ill: Thomas, 1973: 7.

Browne EG. Arabian Medicine. London: Cambridge University Press, 1962.

Clendening L. Source Book of Medical History. New York: Dover, 1960: 87.

Howe GM. A World Geography of Human Disease. London/New York: Academic Press, 1977: 188.

Lendrum FG. Modern Hospital, 1945; 64: 79.

Rosen G. A History of Public Health. New York; MD, 1958: 62.

Sebai ZA. Report on Leprosy in Saudi Arabia. 1973, Unpublished.

World Health Orgnization Expert Committee on Leprosy. World Health Organization Technical Report Series 1970: No. 459.

Hemoglobin and Erythrocytic
Glucose-6-Phosphate Dehydrogenase
Variants Among Selected Tribes
in Western Saudi Arabia

Many studies have been carried out on hemoglobins and glucose -6- phosphate dehydrogenese (G-6-PD) deficiency in Saudi Arabs of the Eastern region bordering the Arabian Gulf.[1, 2, 3, 4, 5, 6, 7, 8, 9, 10, 11] Interest has been generated by a high incidence of both Hb S and G-6-PD deficiency in the oasis of Shia Muslims of the east who represent about 10 percent of the population of Saudi Arabia. No parallel studies have been reported from the western region, although the population of the western region is fairly different from that of the oasis. In the west, the ethnic composition is fairly heterogenous, while the isolated oasis people of the east are ethnically homogenous. Most of the population of Saudi Arabia are Sunni Muslims, however, the oasis people of the east are mainly Shia Muslims who are highly inbred and seldom mix with other Islamic sects. It was thought desirable, therefore, to study the distribution of hemoglobin and G-6-PD variants in the western region and compare findings with those reported from the oasis in the east.

The western region itself is made up of two main areas; Hejaz in the north and Asir mountains in the south. Hejaz is a lowland, with a few scattered hills in which lie the holy cities of Makkah and Medina. Its population is a mixture of various ethnic groups. In addition to the indigenous Arabs there are other immigrant groups who came originally for pilgrimage and settled in Hejaz permanently. This process of immigration to Hejaz has been going on since the beginning of Islam 14 centuries ago.

Asir mountains in the south are 1,200 to 2,100 meters above sea level and until recently were inaccessible. They are inhabited by indigenous Arab tribes whose history goes back several centuries.

Due to the heterogenous nature of the population of the western region our main ojective was therefore to study the distribution of abnormal hemoglobins and G-6-PD variants on a tribal basis. Over a period of six weeks 638 subjects (all Sunni Muslims) from six tribes were tested. In Hejaz, the four tribes of

Harbi, Sahafi, Mograbi and Mowallad, living in the town of Khulais (Figure 11 page 74) and its suburbs were sampled. Two more tribes - Ghamid and Zahran - living around the town of Baljurashi were also sampled (Figure 17 page 152). The results obtained are discussed and compared with findings from the eastern region.

Materials and Methods

A total of 638 subjects from six tribes were tested, 278 males and 60 females from Khulais district in Hejaz and 220 males and 80 females from Baljurashi district in north Asir. In Khulais district (Hejaz) school children from the following four tribes were sampled: (1) Harbi, which indicated several settled Arab Bedouin sub-tribes that live between Makkah and Medina, (2) Sahafi, settled Arab Bedoins, (3) Mograbi, which means Moroccan in Arabic, are settled immigrants who originally came from north Africa; and (4) Mowallad, which literally means half-bred Negroid people, are settled immigrants from Africa. In Baljurashi (Asir), schoolchildren, as well as patients attending Baljurashi Hospital outpatient department, were sampled. Most of these were from two indigenous Arab tribes; (5) Ghamid and (6) Zahran.

Five milliliters of venous blood samples were obtained from a total of 360 subjects for both screening and electrophoretic studies. From the other 278 subjects, fingerprick blood was used for screening purposes only. The venous blood was collected in acid-citrate-dextrose, stored in a portable car refrigerator and flown from Jeddah to Khartoum at wet-ice temperature immediately after completion of collection.

The sickling and G-6-PD deficiency screening tests were performed in the field within two to three hours after collection of venous or fingerprick blood.

The sodium metabisulphite slide test for sickling was done in all 638 subjects. The Brilliant Cresyl Blue (BCB) screening test for G-6-PD deficiency was performed according to Motulsky and Campbell-Kraut[12] in 291 males only. Samples which failed to decolorize the BCB dye up to 180 minute incubation indicated complete deficiency of the enzyme. Intermediate decolorization starting after 60 minutes incubation indicated partial deficiency. Hemoglobin and G-6-PD variants were identified on starch gel electrophoresis using TEB buffer of pH 8.6 following essentially the same method as described by Saha et al. in 1974.[13]

Results and Discussion

Hemoglobin:

The frequency of erythrocyte sickling in six tribes from western Saudi Arabia and the gene frequency of Hb S, in four of these tribes, are presented in Tables 17 and 18 respectively. The results of sickling were identical with that by electrophoresis. The overall frequency of the sickling trait of 2.4 percent compares favorably with 1.1 percent for the western region reported previously by Lehmann et al. in 1963.[14] It is much lower than the overall frequency of 14 percent reported from the eastern region.[15]

In Hejaz, no sickling was found among the two Arab Bedouin tribes of Harbi and Sahafi. Lehmann et al. in 1963[16] also found no sicklers among Bedouins. However, in the other two tribes of Mograbi and Mowallad, the frequency of Hb S was 4.1 and 3.5 percent respectively.

Both Mograbi and Mowallad are newly formed tribes of African origin. It is obvious therefore, that Hb S in Hejaz has been introduced fairly recently, since it is not found in indigenous Bedouins but can be traced to immigrant groups from Africa.

In Asir the frequency of sickling was 4.0 and 2.6 percent respectively in the indigenous Arab tribes of Ghamid and Zahran. Lehmann et al. in 1963[17] reported an incidence of 4 percent in the inhabitants of Najran in southern Asir bordering Yemen. In Yemen itself Hb S is found in some indigenous Arab tribes.[18] Hb S in Asir probably represents part of the overall picture of Hb S in southern Arabia. It could have been introduced from east Africa by the slave trade of the seafaring Arab people of Yemen several thousand years ago. In conclusion, the origin of Hb S in Hejaz and Asir seems to be African. However, it seems that in Hejaz it has been introduced by a different route, across the Red Sea, and much later than in Asir.

Other Hemoglobin Variants:

Only four subjects had elevated hemoglobin A2 which probably represents a low incidence of thalassemia in western Saudi Arabia.

Glucose-6-Phosphate Dehydrogenase Variants:

Results of screening for G-6-PD deficiency and electrophoretic variants in western Saudi Arabia are presented in Tables 19 and 20 respectively. The overall frequency of the complete deficiency of the enzyme in males is 5.8 percent. This is lower than an overall incidence of 13.5 percent in the eastern region.[19] The overall frequencies of GdB and GdA in males were 0.847 and 0.053 respectively.

There are some differences between tribes investigated. In Bedouins and indigenous Arabs (Harbi and Ghamid tribes) both with complete deficiency of the enzyme and the presence of the Gd A+ variant are lower than in African immigrant tribes (Mograbi and Mowallad). In the eastern region the frequency of the Gd A+ variant is 0.091.[20] It is similar to that of Bedouins in the western region. In Ghamid tribe, a new presumptive B slow variant was found. This has been described recently in Sudanese by Saha et al. in 1978[21] and given the trivial name Gd Khartoum.

Table 17. Incidence of Erythrocyte Sickling in Western Saudi Arabia.

Tribe	Number Tested	Number with Sickling	Frequencey of Sickling (%)
Harbi	88	––	––
Sahafi	54	––	––
Mograbi	73	3	4.1
Mowallad	57	2	3.5
Ghamid	177	7	4.0

Zahran	114	3	2.6
Others	75	--	--
Total	638	15	2.4

Table 18. Hemoglobin Types in Western Saudi Arabia.

Tribe	Number Tested	Hemoglobin No. Type	Gene Frequency of Hb S (%)
Harbi	75	75 - A	--
Mograbi	70	67 - A	
		3 - AS	2.1
Mowallad	51	49 - A	
		2 - AS	2.0
Ghamid	62	57 - A	
		4 - AS	3.2
		1 - A2	
Others	76	71 - A	
		2 - AS*	1.3
		3 - A2	
Total	334	319 - A	
		11 - AS	1.6
		4 - A2	

Both Hb As from Zahran tribe (see Table).

Table 19 Glucose-6-Phosphate Dehydrogenase Deficiency in Western Saudi Arabia (ACB Dye Decolorization).

Tribe	Number Tested (All males)	Number with Complete Deficiency	Number with Partial Deficiency	Frequency %
Herbi	61	1	6	9.8
Mograbi	53	4	2	11.3
Mowallad	44	3	5	18.2
Ghamid- -	80	6	3	11.3
Others	53	3	7	18.9
Total	291	17	22	13.4

In subjects with G-6-PD deficiency, it could not be determined whether the deficiency is of A–– or Mediterranean variants for non-availability of white cells or family data and these have been designated Gd––. The frequencies of Gd–– were higher in Mograbi and Mowallad than among Bedouins and indigenous Arabs. However, since a high incidence of A+ variant was found in both Mograbi and Mowallad tribes, it seems probable that the deficiency is due to the Negro A–– variant. This does not exclude the Mediterranean variant since it has been reported in Bedouins in the eastern region.[22]

Comparison of Results of Screening and Electrophoresis for G-6-PD Deficiency:

In subjects in whom both tests have been performed there was some disparity in results (Table 21). There were six in 243 subjects in whom the deficiency had been detected by electrophoresis but were positive on screening. This is probably due to storage effects on enzyme activity. However, there were six out of 12 subjects who were negative on screening but positve (GdB +) on electrophoresis.

Table 20. Glucose-6-Phosphate Dehydrogenase Variants (Electrophoretic) in Western Saudi Arabia.

Tribe	Number Tested (all Males)	Variants B+	A+	B slow	Difficient Gd-
Harbi	59	57 (0.966)	1 (0.017)	--	1 (0.017)
Mograbi	53	41 (0.773)	8 (0.151)	--	4 (0.075)
Mowallad	47	38 (0.809)	4 (0.085)	1 (0.021)	4 (0.085)
Ghamid	62	48 (0.774)	1 (0.016)	10 (0.161)	3 (0.048)
Others	60	54 (0.900)	1 (0.017)	2 (0.033)	3 (0.050)
Total	281	238 (0.847)	15 (0.053)	13 (0.046)	15 (0.053)

Figures in parenthesis denote frequencies.

Similar discrepancy between assay and gel electrophoresis has been reported by Nance in 1977[23] in six samples as Gd A + on electrophoresis and deficient on assay. It is possible that on screening another enzyme deficiency is involved in the hexose-monophosphate shunt pathway. From 19 subjects with partial deficiency, only three were negative on electrophoresis.

Table 21. Brilliant Cresyl Blue Screening and Electrophoresis for Glucose-6-Phosphate Dehydrogenase.

BCB Screening	Number Tested	Electrophoresis Positive	Defficient
Positive	243	237	6
Negative (Complete deficiency)	12	6	6
Negative (Partial deficiency)	19	16	3
Total	274	259	15

Conclusion

The pattern of distribution of Hb S and G-6-PD variants in western Saudi Arabia is similar to that in surrounding countries,[24] but with some local tribal variations which distinguished three groups from each other. (1) In Bedouins of Hejaz (Harbi and Sahafi tribes) there was no sickling and a low frequency of both G-6-PD deficiency and the African gene Gd A+. (2) In the newly formed tribes of African origin (Mograbi and Mowallad) the frequencies of Hb S, G-6-PD deficiency and the Gd A+ variant were higher than in the first group. (3) In Ghamid and Zahran, indigenous Bedouin Arabs of Asir, Hb S frequency was higher than that of Bedouins in Hejaz, but similar to that in the second group. In Ghamid, G-6-PD deficiency and the Gd A+ variant were low in frequency. A new B slow G-6-PD variant was common among the Ghamid.

When results were compared with the findings from the eastern region of Saudi Arabia, it was clear that the populations in this series are fairly different from those in the east. In the east, the Shia Muslims of the Oasis have high incidence of both Hb S (25 percent) and G-6-PD deficiency (13 percent).[25,26] Gelpi in 1965[27] concluded that the Shia Muslims are a distinct minority group in whom there is probably a phenomenon of genetic drift. Similar pockets of high Hb S have been reported previously in India.[28] Our results confirmed the high incidence of Hb S and G-6-PD deficiency in the oais people of the east represents isolated pockets of these genes.

BIBLIOGRAPHY

1. Lehmann H, Maranjian G, Mourant AE. Nature. London, 1963: 198: 492.

2. Maranjian G, Ikin EW, Mourant AE, Lehmann H. Human Biology 1966; 38: 394.

3. Gelpi AP. Blood; 1965: 25: 486.

4. Gelpi AP. Journal of Pediatrics; 1967a: 71: 138.

5. Gelpi AP. Bulletin of the World Health Organization; 1967b: 37: 539.

6. Gelpi AP. Acta Haematologica; 1970: 43: 89.

7. Gelpi AP. King MC. Hum. Hared. 1977: 27: 285.

8. Perrine RP. American Journal of Medicine 1973; 54: 327.

9. Perrine RP, John P. American Journal of Obstetrics and Gynaecology 1974: 118: 29.

10. Pembrey ME, Weatherall DJ, Clegg JB, Bunch C, Perrine RP. British Journal of Haematology 1975: 29: 221.

11. McNeil JR. Journal of the Medical Association of Thailand 1971: 54: 153.

12. Motulsky AG, Campbell-Kraut JM. Proceedings of Conference on Genetic Polymorphism and Geographic Variation in Disease. New York: Grune and Stratton, 1961.

13. Saha N, Kirk RL, Shanbhag S, Joshi SH, Bhatia HM. Hum. Hared. 1974: 24: 198.

14. Lehmann H, Maranjian G, Mourant AE. Nature. London, 1963: 198: 492.

15. Gelpi AP. Journal of Pediatrics; 1967a: 71: 138.

16. Lehmann H. Maranjian G. Mourant AE. Nature. London, 1963: 198: 492.

17. Lehmann H, Maranjian G, Mourant AE. Nature. London, 1963: 198: 492.

18. Lehmann H, Huntsman RG. Man's Haemoglobin. Oxford: North Holland Publishing Company, Amsterdam, 1974.

19. Gelpi AP. Blood, 1965: 25: 486.

20. Gelpi AP, King MC. Hum. Hared. 1977: 27: 285.

21. Saha N, Samuel APW, Ahmed MA, Abdulla HA, Gaddoura EMG. Annals of Human Biology 1978.

22. Gelpi AP, King MC. Hum. Hared. 1977: 27: 285.

23. Nance WE. American Journal of Human Genetics 1977: 29: 537.

24. Lehmann H, Huntsman RG. Man's Haemoglobin. Oxford: North Holland Publishing Company, Amsterdam, 1974.

25. Lehmann H. Maranjian G, Mourant AE. Nature. London, 1963: 198: 492.

26. Gelpi AP. Bulletin of the World Organization; 1967b: 37: 539.

27. Gelpi AP. Blood; 1965; 25:486.

28. Saha N, Banerjee B. Acta. Genet. Med. Gemmellol. 1973; 22: 117.

Chapter V

HEALTH SERVICES AND HEALTH MANPOWER DEVELOPMENT

- Health Manpower: The Problem Facing Saudi Arabia

- Health Manpower in Qasim Region

- A Study of Three Rural Health Centers

- Planning for Primary Health Care in Turaba

- The Role of the Hospitals in Training Professionals in Primary Health Care

- Medical Education: Which Way Forward?

- A New Faculty of Medicine at Abha

- Why Should We Follow Western Style Medical Education? (Arabic)

- Why Don't We Teach Medicine in Arabic? (Arabic)

Health Manpower: The Problem Facing Saudi Arabia

The Kingdom of Saudi Arabia has experienced rapid economic growth since the inception of the first Five-year plan in 1970. The health service system has expanded significantly over the last 10 years, bringing a large influx of expatriate health workers into the Kingdom with different social, cultural and educational backgrounds. Probably the biggest problem is how to utilize at an optimum level the continuously increasing number of personnel with their vastly different backgrounds. An even greater challenge in planning for health manpower in Saudi Arabia is the lack of adequate information in the area of health manpower itself.

This study was carried out in 1982 with the collaboration of the Ministry of Health and the Ministry of Planning. Its objective was to provide an outline of health manpower in Saudi Arabia with particular emphasis on physicians and health assistants, and to give some suggestions for its development.

By 1984, many changes have occurred in the health manpower situation including numbers, distribution and utilization, but no reliable or complete information is available. We intend to leave the 1982 study as it is and add a follow-up comment on the recent developments. In Volume II of the book, we will discuss the propects of health manpower based on a field survey.

The potential for improvement in health manpower in Saudi Arabia is unique because of the available resources and willingness of the authorities to promote its development.

Health Manpower: The Present Situation

In 1981 there were 5,712 physicians working in Saudi Arabia, of whom 60 percent were general practitioners. The remainder were specialists with two to four years of postgraduate training. There is an uneven urban-rural distribution of the physicians in that almost 85 percent work in the 96 hospitals and more than 400 private clinics located in the cities where only 40 percent of the population live. The rest work in 380 health centers located mostly in rural communities. Only 756 (10 percent) of the physicians were Saudi nationals. As is true in most countries, physicians working in Saudi Arabia have been trained principally in clinically oriented, hospital-based institutions which emphasize the physician-patient relationship. Many are not adequately aware of the ecology of prevalent disease and of the socioeconomic and cultural background of Saudi society.

There are 12,800 health assistants in Saudi Arabia (1980) of whom 21 percent are Saudis. The term 'health assistant' includes all personnel who have been trained for two to four years (sometimes more) in a health career, following six to 12 years of elementary education. It therefore includes nurses and all paramedics working in areas such as laboratories, radiology, anesthesiology, statistics, health inspection, etc. There is unfortunately no current information on their present distribution within the Kingdom.

In the country there are four health institutes for male health assistants and seven nursing schools for females. Students are accepted after nine years of basic education and are trained for two to three years. After graduation, health assistants typically become employed in the government health sectors and prefer to work in city hospitals. Females, as a rule, do not yet occupy positions in primary health care units.

The training programs for health assistants face difficulties. The health institutes together can enroll up to 400 new students per year, and the nursing schools up to 450. However, from the foundation of the first health institute in 1958 and the first nursing school in 1961, up to 1979 the number of graduates was only 2,484 health assistants and 535 female nurses. Attracting young Saudis to training programs in paramedical careers is not easy, as both boys and girls prefer to complete secondary school education and then enter the universities, which are free for all Saudis, both male and female. Such an education provides prestige and more promising career prospects. Few of those who seek professional training select nursing or health care as their first choice, as other careers offer higher financial rewards and greater prestige.

In 1980 there were only 280 dentists in the Kingdom (three dentists per 10,000 people) of whom 11 percent were Saudis. While the College of Dentistry (established in 1975) will help to change this in the future, there are two other problems - inadequate preventive orientation of the dentists and an inadequate number of dental assistants. The situation is better in pharmacy, there being 860 pharmacists in the country, of whom half are Saudis. Since the establishment of the Faculty of Pharmacy of King Saud University in 1959, there have been 464 graduates - 65 percent of them Saudis. Nevertheless like the medical faculties, the Faculty of Pharmacy needs to become more relevant to the health needs of the country.

The lack of effective management is a serious deficiency in the delivery of health services in all developing countries, and Saudi Arabia is no exception. Many present top-level managers need reorientation programs in public health administration and health planning, programming and evaluation. A new generation of young Saudis needs to be trained in health management at all levels to cope with the rapid expansion of the health services system.

Health Manpower: The Future (1990)

This is a preliminary attempt to outline possible alternatives for health manpower development by 1990. It is a short period for planning, but it has been arbitrarily chosen because of the lack of adequate data and the difficulties in predicting the many variables. When preparing a health manpower plan it is important to have available statistical data such as population dynamics, morbidity and mortality rates as well as reliable information about the social and organizational changes.

In Saudi Arabia, unfortunately, little of the relevant data is available and therefore approaches to planning must be more pragmatic. In 1981 the population of Saudi Arabia was estimated to be approximately 8.8 million and the projection for the target years, 1990 is 10.7 million. The following has been limited to the requirements for physicians and health assistants. Further work is needed to draw up a comprehensive plan for all health manpower development.

Table 1 shows the number of physicians and health assistants (Saudis and total) for the year 1981 and two possible action plans for the year 1990.

Table 1. Health Manpower in Saudi Arabia: in 1981 and Two Alternative Plans for 1990.

	1981	Alternative Plan for 1990	
		1.	**2.**
Population (millions)	8.8	10.7	10.7
No. of physicians	5,712	8,900	10,700
Population per physician	1,660	1,200	1,000
No. of Saudi physicians	576 (10%)	4,450 (50%)	7,500 (70%)
No. of health assistants	12,800	35,600	64,200
Health assistants per physician	2.4	4	6
No. of Saudi health assistants	2,700 (21%)	17,800 (50%)	45,000 (70%)

"Alternative 1" calls for a ratio of one physician to 1,200 population. The figure allows for an average of five outpatient visits per person per year if a comprehensive health team approach is used, and 160 admissions per 1,000 population per year with an average hospital stay of eight days. Of the 8,900 physicians, 50 percent will be Saudis. On the assumption that 3,130 physicians will graduate from the four medical schools in Saudi Arabia in the period 1981-1990 and a further 1,180 overseas, and taking into account the 576 Saudi physicians already working in the Kingdom, there will be sufficient Saudi physicians in 1990 to meet 50 percent of the needs projected in "Alternative 1," even allowing for 10 percent attrition over the period. By extrapolation it can be estimated that by the year 2,000 there will be 8,535 Saudi physicians, i.e. 73 percent of the total of required physicians if the ratio of one physician to 1,200 population is to be maintained. Therefore in term of physicians "Alternative 1" seems realistic and attainable.

"Alternative 2" on the other hand, calls for a ratio of one physician to 1,000 inhabitants. It looks more appealing and prestigious, but it is more expensive, difficult to attain and possibly would turn out to be less productive, as physicians would perform the tasks of paramedics with less satisfaction and efficiency. Studies indicate that there is no positive correlation between increasing the number of physicians and hospitals, and the standard of health care delivered (Duque 1978).

The main objective of the health service system, as stated in the Third Development Plan, is to improve the health status of the people of Saudi Arabia. At the top of the list of strategies necessary to achieve this goal is the expansion of preventive health programs including vaccination, health sanitation, health education, early detection of disease, and maternal and child health, all of which need to be delivered through primary care units (Ministry of Planning, Saudi Arabia 1981). If this comprehensive health care program is to be achieved, the medical education programs of the four Saudi faculties of medicine will have to demonstrate more clearly their commitment to meeting the real needs of the family and the community.

At present only five of the 576 Saudi physicians in the country are trained in public health. In our opinion, by 1990 some 20 percent of all physicians should be in training or have complete training in the areas of public health and family and community medicine. In the United States, about 25 percent of newly graduated physicians from many faculties of medicine choose family medicine as a specialty. An analysis of residencies by specialty in the United States in 1979 showed that out of 26 specialties available, family medicine ranked second in popularity after internal medicine (American Medical Association 1980). In Saudi Arabia and other Gulf countries we must place more emphasis on this subject.

A postgraduate institute of family and community medicine should be established. This institute must not merely replicate similar establishments in the western countries, but should be carefully planned to meet the health needs of Saudi Arabia and neighboring countries. The institute would develop postgraduate training and research programs in the area of family medicine for practicing physicians, and community medicine for health planners, administrators, managers and professionals in preventive medicine.

An essential point to emphasize is that in Saudi Arabia, health problems must be tackled by health teams. Although in the future we will have a significant number of Saudi physicians, there will remain a serious shortage of Saudi health assistants. "Alternative 1" for 1990 calls for 17,800 Saudi health assistants (60 percent males).

If we assume that the four health institutes and seven nursing schools continue to graduate students at the present level, by 1990 there will be a total of 5,847 Saudi health assistants employed (if one allows for a 15 percent attrition rate) and of these, 74 percent will be males. This total is only 16 percent of the total number of health assistants proposed for 1990 in "Alternative 1." In order to produce the additional 6,366 male health assistants and 5,607 female health assistants, 15 health institutes and 65 nursing schools would have to be established.

This ambitious suggestion is neither practical nor feasible and other approaches should be given serious consideration. These include an increase in enrollment in the existing institutions and a reduction in the attrition rate, the creation of health assistant training programs in selected hospitals and primary care units, the training of community health workers (successful programs can be found in Yemen and Sudan), an extension of the target date of the plan from 1990 or 1995, or a combination of all three.

Summary and Conclusion

The following features characterize health personnel in the Kingdom today:

1. Only 10 percent of the physicians and 21 percent of the health assistants in Saudi Arabia are Saudis. This situation leads to problems of communication and effectiveness.

2. The majority of the health personnel lack the proper orientation towards the particular needs of the country.

3. The lack of sufficient managerial personnel at all levels is a limiting factor in the operation and expansion of the health services system.

4. There is an uneven urban-rural distribution of health personnel.

Recommendations for the future include the following:

1. Special importance should be given to teacher training and to establishing programs for continuing education of all health personnel.

2. The prospect of producing a sufficient number of appropriately trained Saudi health assistants is poor, and the situation deserves thoughtful and decisive consideration by the health authorities and educational institutes.

3. A postgraduate institute of family and community medicine should be established.

4. Curative, promotive and preventive aspects of health services should be integrated.

5. The organization and management of health services should be regionalized and decentralized.

6. Comprehensive analytic studies in the area of health services/health manpower development should be carried out.

Follow-up Comments

There is no accurate or complete data on health manpower in the health sector. Data is under collection now by the Ministry of Health and the Ministry of Planning. A field survey, sponsored by the Saudi Arabian National Center for Science and Technology (SANCST) is planned to cover the area of health manpower and the results will be published in the second volume of this book.

There are indications of progress in the last few years.

The three faculties of medicine in Riyadh, Jeddah and Dammam have produced collectively 244 Saudi doctors since their establishments (131 male and 113 female). The almost equal ratio of males to females requires a close inspection of its implications on the future of the health services system. The faculty of medicine at Abha will produce its first batch of graduates in 1988. The target of producing about 3,500 Saudi physicians from the four faculties of medicine in the Kingdom by 1990 seems to be feasible. At present there is a continuous assessment of the curriculae of the faculties of medicine and efforts are being made to improve the objectives and methods of education.

Postgraduate education programs have already started in various clinical and academic fields. The Arab Boards for Medical Specializations approved all the universities' hospitals for residency programs in medicine, surgery, pediatrics and gynaecology and obstetrics. The residency program in family and community medicine is to be established in King Faisal University.

The Faculty of Dentistry at King Saud University in Riyadh has 156 male students and 201 female students. Since 1981 this faculty has produced 37 dentists, all Saudi. Another faculty of dentistry is planned at King Abdul Aziz University in Jeddah.

The Faculty of Pharmacy has 365 students, 211 Saudi and 154 non-Saudi. The total number of graduates since its establishment in 1959 is 533 (40 percent were non-Saudis). There is a need to improve the prospects of future careers for pharmacists in order to attract Saudi applicants to the faculty. A second faculty of pharmacy is under planning at King Abdulaziz University in Jeddah.

Other medical institutions, such as the faculties of allied health sciences in Riyadh and Jeddah, and the faculty of veterinary medicine in Al Ahsa are also recording progress in numbers of students and curriculum development.

Health Institutes

Recently the title of the nursing schools has been changed to Health Institutes for females. Table (2) shows the development of health institutes for males and females in the period 1980-1984.

Table 2. Development of Health Institutes for Males and Females 1980- 1984.

	MALES		FEMALES	
	1980	1984	1980	1984
Number of institutes	4	12	7	14
Total number of graduates since establishement	2484	3129	535	758

In conclusion, health manpower is progressing steadily. This is especially true of the number of Saudi physicians. For other members of the health team, although the number of training institutes has increased, there is still a great need to attract more applicants to the field. Curriculum development is in progress.

The ultimate goal should be to produce adequate numbers of the various members of the health team whose training is suitable for the present and future needs of the country. This should be the first priority in the planning of health development in Saudi Arabia.

Recommended Literature

1. American Medical Association. Director of Residency Training Programs, 1980; AMA, Chicago.

2. Duque LF. An Integrated Approach: The Latin-American Experience. WHO/EMRO Technical Publication 1978; 1:143

3. Ministry of Planning, Saudi Arabia. Third Development Plan (1980-1985). 1981; 286.

4. Sebai ZA. The Health of the Family in a Changing Arabia: A Case Study of Primary Health Care. Jeddah: Tihama Publications, 1983; 19-22.

5. Sebai ZA, Baker TD. Projected Needs of Health Manpower in Saudi Arabia, 1974-90. Medical Education 1976: 10, 359-361.

Health Manpower Study In Qasim Region

This study of health manpower in Qasim was conducted in 1980 as part of a general survey in Qasim region (p. 99). It discusses some attributes of health personnel and the problems they face. It also provides suggestions for improvement. It is hoped that the study will contribute to the development of health services in the region.

The Qasim region has a population of 370,000. It is mostly rural and its economy depends on agriculture and government employment. There are five hospitals (with a total of 459 beds), 42 health centers and 28 health dispensaries. Altogether there are 1,218 health personnel, 95 percent of whom work in the Ministry of Health sector. The rest work in the school health department and in the municipality. There are a few physicians who run private practices in the main cities.

A sample of 20 percent of the total health personnel was selected at random to represent the various categories working in different health units.

A structured questionnaire was prepared to collect the following information on each respondent: place of work, sex, nationality, nature of work, basic education and training (including past experience), problems encountered at work and suggestions for improvement. The pre-coded questionnaires were filled in by the health personnel in their offices and clinics after a brief introduction by the investigators. The collected data was then tabulated and analyzed. The health personnel were classified into four groups: physicians, nurses, technical assistants and administrative staff.[1] The technical assistants include laboratory, and X-ray technicians, statistical analysts, health inspectors, etc. Sometimes nurses and technical assistants are referred to as one category - "health assistants."

Results and Discussions

Overall Distribution of Health Manpower in Qasim.

In Qasim there are 264 physicians and 847 health assistants* (nurses and technical assistants) serving 370,000 inhabitants. The ratio of physicians to population in Qasim is one to 1,400 (in Saudi Arabia as a whole it is one to 1,500). There are 3.2 health assistants for one physician (2.8 throughout Saudi Arabia). Although the people in Qasim are predominantly rural, 70 percent of the health personnel work in the five hospitals located in the three main cities (Table 3).

Altogether 54 percent of the work force is male (Table 4). Out of 264 physicians there are only two Saudis (occupying the highest administrative positions). None of the 394 female nurses are Saudi.

Characteristics of the Sample.

Our sample included 249 health personnel (64 physicians, 109 nurses, 58 technical assistants and 18 administrative staff). They constitute 20 percent of the total number of health workers.

Nationalities: Table 5 summarizes the distibution of a sample by nationality. The Qasim region relies heavily on Egyptian physicians - about 70 percent of the total. Nurses used to be recruited from Egypt and other Arab states, but lately an increasing number of nurses have been recruited from the Philippines (44 percent of the nursing staff). This is mainly because the Gulf countries have exhausted the supply of Egyptian nurses. Thirty-three percent of the technical assistants are also from the Philippines. This brings to mind the difficulty of communication due to language and cultural barriers. Most of the nurses and technical assistants are young and single and are living in very conservative communities.

---

*   In addition there are a few health professionals such as pharmacists.

About half the health personnel are under the age of 30 years (11 percent are over 40). This indicates that most recruits have recently completed training.

Basic education and training (Table 6).

Because of the differences among different countries in the basic education and period of training required for the health assistants, we chose to consider the total number of years spent on basic education and training together under the term "basic education and training."

Forty-one percent of the physicians were reported as specialists (mostly with one-to-two year diploma courses). More than half the health assistants, primarily Filipinos, had 15 to 16 years of basic education and training. Other nationalities were less qualified than the Filipinos. All the Saudi administrative staff had less than secondary education (12 years of education) and no one in the administration had had any formal training in management. The gap between the education and training of the technical staff and the administrative staff is wide. The main bottle-neck of health services delivery systems in developing countries is in management and administration.

Table 3. Percentage Distribution of Health Personnel in Qasim According to Place of Work (Total Number 1,218).

Health Personnel	Total No.	Percentage Working in	
		Hospitals	Others Units*
Physicians	264	67	33
Nurses	464	65	35
Technical assistants	383	67	33
Administrative staff	107	93	7
Total	1,218	70	30

* Including dispensaries, health centers and other types of health service units.

Table 4. Percentage Distribution of Health Personnel According to Sex (Total Number 1,218).

Health Personnel	MALE		FEMALE	
	No.	%	No.	%
Physicians	198	75	66	25
Nurses	70	15	394	85
Technical assistants	283	74	100	26
Administrative staff	107	100	0	0
Total	658	54	560	46

Table 5. Percentage Distribution of Health Personnel in the Sample According to Nationality (Total Number 249).

Health Personnel				Nationality		
	No.	Saudi	Egyptian	Other Arabs	Pakistani /Indian	Filipino
Physicans	64	0	70	8	11	11
Nurses	109	3	40	6	7	44
Technical assts.	58	12	22	19	14	33
Administrators	18	94	6	0	0	0

Table 6. Percentage Distribution of Health Personnel in the Sample According to Basic Education and Training in Years (Total Number 249).

Health Personnel	No.	Duration of (%) Education and Training in Years.			
		-12	12-14	15-16	16+
Physicians	64				100
Nurses	109	9	37	50	4
Technical assts.	58	7	23	65	5
Administrators	18	50	39	5	6

Few of the personnel had been through any training program after completing their basic training. Eighteen percent of the general physicians and 11 percent of the health assistants reported such supervised training in a hospital or health center. Only three percent of the personnel had been through a continuing education program which included seminars or conferences.

A substantial number of the expatriate workers were new arrivals in Qasim; about 37 percent of them had worked there for only one year or less. This is attributed to both the high turnover and the continuous expansion of health services. No one in the sample population had received any orientation program on the health situation in Saudi Arabia or Qasim.

Orientation programs at the beginning of assignments for expatriates who have been trained in circumstances different from those of Saudi Arabia would be of great value in introducing them to the type of health problems and their etiology in the country. The same would apply to inservice training and continuing education programs for physicians, health assistants and administrators. This would ultimately lead to better productivity and effectiveness. Arabic language courses are essential for non-Arabic speaking personnel.

Problems Encountered by the Health Personnel and Their Suggestions for Improvement

The respondents were asked to state the problems they face at work as well as suggestions for improving their working conditions. A summary of problems encountered by the respondents is given in Table 7. Few of the administrative staff responded to the questions and they are excluded from the table.

The most serious complaints concerned (a) lack of facilities and equipment, (b) communication barriers, and (c) high work load. The explanations are:

(a) Although the Ministry of Health is going through a process of administrative reform, especially regarding regionalization of health services, many decisions are still taken at a central level in Riyadh. This hinders the process of purchasing, distribution, maintenance and utilization of equipment and supplies.

Table 7. Order of Major Problems Encountered at Work by the Type of Health Personnel (1 = High, 3 = Low, –– = Occasionally Mentioned).

Problems	Respondents		
	Physicians	Nurses	Technical Assistants
Lack of facilities and equipment	1	3	1
Communication barriers	3	1	1
High work load	1	1	2
Unfair administrative treatment	2	2	2
Poor coordination among staff	––	2	3
Lack of work orientation	––	3	––
Inadequate social life	––	3	3
Lack of health education of the patients	2	3	––

(b) Many health workers, especially the health assistants, are non-Arabs who experience difficulty in language and cultural communication with their patients.

(c) Working hours are nine hours per day. Night shifts and weekend duties are additional burdens. This, in the opinion of the respondents, leaves little time for social life and personal development.

Strangely enough, very few specified their needs for continuing education or orientation programs.

Most of the suggestions for improvement were in direct relation to the problems. The physicians suggested better facilities and equipment, shorter working hours and the need for a health education program for the patients. The suggestions of the nurses included organizing Arabic language courses for non-Arabic speakers, shorter working hours, better management, and orientation programs. For the technical staff, the emphasis was on better facilities, Arabic language courses, improvement of management and inservice training programs. Other individual suggestions were: a better recording system, a medical library, regular staff meetings, organized social activities and improving housing conditions.

Those who worked in health centers and dispensaries in the rural areas faced common problems in the lack of proper social life and of adequate facilities for shopping, banking and schools for their children.

From general discussions with physicians another problem was apparent, though not shown in their responses to the questionnaire, and that was the lack of job satisfaction. The physician in his outpatient clinic may handle over 100 patients per day. In many instances he spends not more than two minutes per patient.

Conclusions and Recommendations

This study identified various attributes of the health workers in the Qasim region and to provide basic information to assist in better planning.

The study showed that: (1) the distribution of health personnel between urban and rural units in Qasim was uneven, (2) health services were heavily dependent on expatriate personnel, (3) health services personnel had completed basic training but lacked experience in the needs of the region, (4) health personnel had no means of finding out about new developments in medical knowledge, (5) the administrative staff was not sufficiently educated and trained.

The situation could be improved by organizing orientation programs for newcomers, continuing education courses, inservice training for all categories which would include administrators, and regular Arabic language courses.

In order to keep abreast of relevant new developments in medical knowledge, libraries should be established. These would benefit health personnel as a whole and raise the standard of health services. Better facilities and living conditions should be provided for personnel.

If a system of record-keeping, patient screening and management reform were introduced, it would minimize the work load and give more time to personnel for personal development and innovative actions. The system should be comprehensive (curative, preventive and promotive).

It was clear that all health personnel, especially the director of the regional services and his assistant, were deeply interested in determining the problems and in studying how to improve the situation. Futher studies are needed to analyze the present function of health manpower and of the health services sytem. Any action in the future should be followed up, monitored and evaluated with feedback on planning and implementation.

A Study of Three Rural Health Centers

The main objective of this study is to draw a profile of the function of three rural health centers in Saudi Arabia in Khulais, Wadiyen and Tamnia. These centers are not representative of the health centers in the country, but nevertheless do not differ much from others.

The three health centers have been studied on different occasions. The study of Khulais and Tamnia centers was part of a supervised training program for fourth-year medical students carried out in the fall of 1977 and 1979. The Wadiyen study was part of a physician training program in community medicine conducted in the summer of 1978. All the programs were organized by the Community Medicine Department, King Saud Faculty of Medicine, in collaboration with the Ministry of Health.

A new trend in health care has developed in the late 1970s in Saudi Arabia. It emphasizes primary health care, health manpower development and decentralization of health services, a development which might show results in the near future. It would be of interest to re-evaluate the health center activities periodically to assess any new developments.

The Communities

Khulais community is a rural area in western Saudi Arabia with a population of 18,000 and is composed of a small town, Khulais, and six clusters of villages. Khulais town, where the health center is located, is connected by 90 kilometers of asphalted road to Jeddah, the main port of Saudi Arabia.

Wadiyen and Tamnia are two rural communities in the southwest (30 kilometers apart), each approximately 40 kilometers from Abha, the capital of the region. Wadiyen is comprised of a group of small villages whose estimated population is 3,700. Tamnia community has a population of 2,050 distributed through nine small villages (ranging from 171 to 713 inhabitants per village).

There are some common features in the three communities. The major occupations of the people are farming, government employment and trading. Most of the adults are semi-literate, whereas the young boys and girls pursue their education in recently established schools.

The health problems in the three communities are not much different from other rural communities. They are mainly due to inadequate sanitation and lack of health education. Diarrhea and respiratory infections are leading causes of morbidity among young children. The infant mortality rate is estimated at 120 per thousand live births. Schistosomiasis is endemic in Khulais. The demands of the villagers for health services, as shown in other studies,[1] are for hospitals, more physicians, X-ray machinery, and injections, which are quite different from their actual health needs.

The health centers are the first point of contact for the villagers. However, the distance from the city is not a hindrance to some people, especially male adults, seeking health services in the city hospitals.

The Three Health Centers

The three health centers are located in rented buildings. They are open for eight hours daily (five and a half days a week). Only in Khulais are there laboratory and X-ray facilities, but these are not functioning yet. Each health center is staffed by a physician and four to six health assistants: pharmacy, laboratory and X-ray assistants and nurses (Table 8), all non-Saudis. This reflects not only the shortage of Saudi health personnel, but also their uneven urban-rural distribution.

The Activities of the Health Centers may be divided into curative and preventive health services.

Curative Services

These are outpatient health services. The daily attendance at the three centers is shown in Table 8. Patients under the age of five years constituted 18 percent of the total. The male to female ratio was 1.6:1. The rate of population attendance is influenced by various factors including seasonal variations, tribal disputes and distances from the center.

Each patient is seen by the physician. In both Khulais and Wadiyen an observer sitting beside the physician calculated the time spent with each patient. In Khulais the mean for both sexes was 3.1 minutes. In Wadiyen the mean was 2.3 minutes (21 seconds on history taking, 64 seconds on examination and 53 seconds on prescription writing). In the other words, the physicians in Wadiyen and his staff spend about one-and-one-quarter to one-and-one-half hours (15 to 18 percent of their time) every day dealing with outpatients.

Table 8. Population of the Three Communities, Attendance and Staff of the Health Centers.

Health Center	Estimated Population	No.	%	Physicians	Health assistants
		Daily Attendance		**Staff**	
Khulais	1800	136	0.8	1	6
Wadiyen	3,700	36	1.0	1	5
Tamnia	2,050	48	2.3	1	4

Sixteen patients were interviewed after they were discharged from the outpatient department in Wadiyen health center. Of these, four knew their diagnosis and five knew how to use the medicine as prescribed. These figures suggest a failure to absorb the information given to them by their doctor relating to their diagnosis and management.

Diagnosis is made according to the "body system." It is written on a prescription sheet or in a log book. At the end of each month the physician completes a monthly form designed by the Ministry of Health, and sends it to the regional office. Excerpts from a monthly form from the Tamnia health center are shown in Table 9.

Table 9. Excerpt of a Monthly Report of Cases Seen in Tamnia Health Center.

Disease	Out-patient visits			
	Men	Women	Children	Total
Infections	0	0	0	0
Cardiovascular diseases	104	87	44	235
Chest diseases	340	270	110	720
Gastrointestinal diseases	351	214	117	682
Genitourinary diseases	177	108	43	328
Obstetrics/Gynaecology	0	38	0	38

Prescriptions made out during a single day at Khulais center showed that tonics accounted for nearly one-third of the 288 items dispensed. Of the 206 active preparations prescribed, 62 (30 percent) were antibiotics and 49 (24 percent) were antipyretics/analgesics. Forty-five percent of the analgesics and antirheumatics and 18 percent of antibiotics (including chloramphenicol for children) were given in injection form (injections are in great demand). A patient may receive an injection of antibiotics and a three day supply of capsules which he might discard or use irregularly. The analysis of a list of prescriptions made over a month in Wadiyen and Tamnia is not very different from that in Khulais. Such indiscriminate usage of antibiotics and other active drugs by the patients may do more harm than good.

Preventive Services

Practically no organized preventive health services are being offered by the health centers.

Only at Khulais health center have vaccinations been given during the last year as shown in Table 10. In Wadiyen and Tamnia no vaccinations were given in the last one-and-one-half years and 10 years respectively (the length of time during which the two physicians had been there).

Table 10. Vaccines Given at Khulais Health Center, from April to April 1977.

Antigen	No. Vaccinated
DPT. 1st dose	465
2nd dose	194
3rd dose	47
Polio: 1st dose	207
2nd dose	1
3rd dose	0
Smallpox	32
Cholera	122
Typhoid	19

An analysis of the recorded vaccinations in Khulais has been made. The ages of those vaccinated were recorded for 297 recipients of a first dose of diptheria pertussis tetanus (DPT) vaccine. More than two-thirds of these (201) were at least three years old and only 48 were under the age of one year. The number of second doses of DPT was less than half the number of first doses given and the number of third doses was only about 10 percent of the first dose. Only one child was recorded as having a second dose of polio vaccine and none had a third. If for a population of 18,000, the estimated number of births per year is 810 (birth rate is estimated at 45 per 1,000 per year), only six percent of the children were covered by a complete dosage of DPT and none with polio. Only part of DPT was given at the age of greatest danger.

If we consider the three communities together, with a total population of 23,700, the estimated number of births should be 1,066 per year. The three nurses in the three health centers have attended between them 144 deliveries in one year, amounting to 14 percent of the expected births. The remainder of these deliveries are usually attended by old women in the villages. Registration of births is not complete. No other biomedical statistics were recorded.

A notification of infectious diseases is supposed to be sent each week by all health centers to the regional office. Over the 15 month period, January 1976 to March 1977, Khulais health center reported 418 cases, including pulmonary tuberculosis 204, influenza 66, measles 47, amebic dysentry 28, venereal diseases 3, and non-specific 70. Diagnosis is based on clinical impressions with no means of investigation. Wadiyen Health Center reported 20 cases of infectious disease over a 15 month period, while in Tamnia no report has been sent in the last three years. There is lack of uniformity in the reporting system and minimum supervision or feedback from the regional offices to the health centers.

The three physicians in the health centers have spent three years, 11 years and 10 years respectively in the Kingdom. The last spent the whole of his 10 years in the one community. Only one had participated in a two-week refresher course.

Conclusion

The three health centers in Khulais, Wadiyen and Tamnia rural communities in Saudi Arabia have been studied for their function and efficiency.

The study showed that their main function is to render curative health services to outpatients. The physician spends approximately three minutes with each patient.

The diagnosis is made on clinical presumptions without any diagnostic facilities and is recorded according to the "body system" which gives no clue to the health problems in the community. In many cases medicines are distributed indiscriminately.
Few preventive or promotive health services are provided. In Khulais (population 18,000) 6 percent of the children were covered with a full schedule of DPT, but none with polio. The other two centers gave no vaccinations. Only

14 percent of all births in the three communities were attended by the nurses. Biomedical statistics are not kept.

In conclusion, it can be said that the three health centers are not performing their functions as agencies of health promotion. The reasons are multiple: lack of physicians' undertaking of their role as promoters of the health of the people (basically because their medical training was hospital based and curative oriented), none of the professional staff is Saudi (due to the shortage and unbalanced distribution of Saudis), no adequate planning, supervision and follow up of the functions of the health centers (due to centralization of the organization), and lack of community participation.

Further studies of rural health are needed in order to verify the morbidity and mortality rates, the health needs and demands, and the most appropriate methods of utilizing available and potential resources to upgrade the health of the people.

The progressive attitudes evident in the third five-year plan of the Ministry of Health, starting in 1980, aiming at decentralization and regionalization of health services, strengthening primary health care and developing health manpower, may produce results in a few years. A re-evaluation of the function of the health centers will be of great interest.

Follow-up Comments, 1984

Short visits were paid to Khulais, Tamnia and Wadiyen communities in 1984 to find out if any changes had occurred in the function of the three health centers. The follow-up comments on Khulais Health Center are mentioned under Khulais (pp.85-87). In this section the changes observed in Tamnia and Wadiyen will be discussed, along with comments on the prospects of primary health care in the country.

The Findings

The two health centers in Tamnia and Wadiyen are in the same territory (about 30 kilometers apart). Both health centers have been relocated in new rented buildings which are more spacious than the old ones. Each is run by a physician and three to four health assistant. All personnel are expatriates with the exception of one Saudi pharmacy assistant. The physicians are from Egypt and India and the health assistants are from India, Bangladesh, and the Philippines.

There is no recent census but by estimation the population of Tamnia is 4,000 and of Wadiyen is 5,000.

The function of the two health centers is still curative in nature. Members of the health team do not visit homes except for some normal deliveries attended by the midwives. According to one of the physicians, "In the eight working hours of the day we stay behind our desks treating outpatients." Diagnosis is still made according to the "body system". Thirty-four percent of prescriptions were for antibiotics. Table 11 shows some areas of comparison of the two health centers together in 1978-9 and 1984.

Table 11. Changes in the Two Health Centers in Tamnia and Wadiyen (1978-1984).

	1978	1984
Building	rented houses	rented houses
Laboratory Services	none	exist in Wadiyen
X-ray facilities	none	none
Dental services	none	none
Total population served	5750	9000
Number of physicians	2	2
Number of health assistants	9	7
Total daily attendance (average)	84	115
Pattern of health services	curative	curative
Immunization program	none	exists
Other preventive activities	practically none	practically none

In 1978-1979 no vaccination program was carried out in the two communities, whereas in 1984 a program was in existence. Table 12 shows the number of vaccines given in the last six months to children under 24 months of age in the two communities.

Table 12. Vaccines Given in the Last Six Months to Children 0-24 Months Old.

Vaccine	Tamnia	Wadiyen	Total
Polio and DPT*			
First dose	23	51	74
Second dose	14	41	55
Third dose	12	49	61
Measles	17	43	60
Tetanus	22	51	73
Mumps	—	96	96

*Polio and DPT vaccines are given together at the same time.

The health center in Wadiyen is relatively more active in the immunization program. However, vaccines are only given to children who attend the health centers. There is no follow-up for defaulters. BCG vaccine is not given because, according to the two physicians, it needs special training and none of health assistants are trained for that! The physician in Wadiyen, after a discovery of a few cases of mumps, asked of imam of the mosque to call people after Friday prayers to take their children for immunization. Next morning 93 children were brought in for immunization. This is an indication of how effective the community leaders can be.

If the two communities were taken together with a total population of 9,000 and annual crude birth rates of 45 per 1,000, the estimated number of newborn is 405 per year. If a rate of 15 percent is allowed for stillbirths and child deaths, we still have 690 children below two years of age who need to be immunized (immunization is practically never completed during infancy). Over one year an estimated 122 children received the three doses of polio and DPT, and 120 children received measles vaccine. This means that only 17 percent of the children in Tamnia and Wadiyen have received full coverage of polio, DPT and measles vaccine. Our calculations are rough but still they indicate that some progress has been made since 1978. Nevertheless there is a need for more action, especially at the community level.

Only 19 home deliveries were attended by the two midwives in the two centers over the last six months. Apparently this is far from the optimum in a population with an estimated 405 deliveries per year. The rest of the deliveries are either attended by native women or unreported in hospitals in town.

No other active preventive programs such as school health, health education, maternal and child health, environmental sanitation, control of infectious diseases and nutritional programs practically exist in the two communities.

In Conclusion, five years after our survey in the late 1970's, the two health centers in Tamnia and Wadiyen are still curative oriented with practically no active role in disease prevention.

Which Way Forward?

The unfavorable evaluation of the three health centers in Khulais, Tamnia and Wadiyen in the past and at present leads to the question, "what about the future?"

In any health services system; three components determine the effectiveness of the system.

- The recipients; individuals and communities

- The organizers; high authorities

- The providers; physicians and the members of the health team

The role of individuals and communities in the health services system has already been discussed under "Turaba in the Future."

The trend of the authorities in the Ministry of Health of delegating actions to the regions is very promising. A good example can be found in the Southwestern Region. The recently appointed director of the health services enjoys a wide range of authority. He is a pharmacist and a holder of a masters degree in health administration, an energetic and enthusiastic young administrator who sees his role as a health promoter. This has been reflected in various innovative programs undertaken recently by his office in the region, including training of physicians in oral rehydration therapy, outreach dental services and health education. Luckily, the health authorities encourage other regional directors as well, to be agents for change.

The third component, the physician and his team, is also promising. This is true if special care is given to improving basic medical education and continuing education programs. On several occasions the following question was directed to physicians working in health center: "If you had full authority and almost unlimited resources to promote health in your community, what would you do?" Responses varied. Some physicians could not see the need for any change, but the majority gave constructive ideas such as:

-   extending health care beyond the walls of the center

-   the physician and his team should go out into the community

-   health assistants should be trained to take an active role in health promotion

-   a doctor should see only a limited number of patients (general consensus is 25-30 per day) and the rest of the patients should be screened by health assistants

The responses were not always spelled out in a systematic and methodological way, and community participation was usually missed. However, these concepts could be easily instilled through reorientation courses.

In brief, the health center in Wadiyen, for example, is suitable to start a conceptual model for primary health care based on a scientific approach. The three previously mentioned components for the success of such a project are readily available. The project could be jointly carried out by the Ministry of Health, the Faculty of Medicine at Abha, King Khalid Military Hospital in Khamis Mushyet, other organizations and the community. Some details of the strategy are discussed under "Turaba in the Future." The model could be gradually extended to other areas in the Southwestern Region and throughout the Kingdom.

BIBLIOGRAPHY

1. Sebai ZA. The Health of the Family in a Changing Arabia, 3rd ed. Jeddah: Tihama Publications, 1983.

Planning for Primary Health Care In Turaba

Research in the field of health cannot be an end but rather a means for change. If the previous sections on the situation of primary health care in Turaba, Tamnia, Wadiyen, Khulais and Qasim can work as a stimulant for thinking in the future, this section suggests a guideline for health services development. It is a preliminary plan of action for a primary health care (PHC) model to develop health services in Turaba community (Figure 8, p. 41) by1990.

This guideline is not intended to replace a rational detailed plan, as this is left for further discussion and dynamic thinking. Health planners, health providers, health professionals, technical people and representatives from the community should participate in the planning and implementation of the final program. The proposed PHC plan could be seen as a conceptual model applicable, after modification, to other communities in Saudi Arabia and possibly abroad. Continuous evaluation and feedback should be integral parts of its implementation.

The Plan of Action

1. Objectives

    - To provide a comprehensive health care program (curative, preventive and promotive) design to (a) reduce morbidity and mortality and (b) improve the health status of the people.

    - To provide training and research opportunities for health personnel.

2. Functions

    - The provision of comprehensive and integrated health services to individuals, families and the community, including curative services, health education, environmental sanitation, maternal and child health, nutrition, immunization and mental health.

    - Services should be carried out with full participation of the community in identifying the problems, planning and programming, implementation, follow-up and evaluation. This would develop an appreciation for the health services, better communication and understanding of the local values, self-reliance and mobilization of resources.

    - Training programs at both undergraduate and postgraduate levels of medical students, doctors, planners, administrators and other health workers would enhance future developments.

    - Collection of base-line data and carrying out applied research for better understanding of the health problems and their ecological background, and to search for proper solutions.

3. Basic Considerations

    People:

- There is no up-to-date census or demographic data available. The population is estimated at 45,000; 20 percent are Bedouins, the annual population growth is about 3.6 percent. The settlement of the Bedouins, migration to the cities and importation of foreign laborers is a continuing process. Children below 15 years of age constitute 40 percent of the population.

- The basic health problems are related to inadequate sanitation, lack of health education and infectious diseases.

- Turaba is developing socioeconomically. This will lead to a change in lifestyle, better housing, nutrition and education.

Primary Health Care:

- Primary health care is neither a second class solution for poor countries nor a cheap method to apply. It is rather the challenge of meeting the basic and essential needs and demands of the people in an integrated and comprehensive way.

- All member states of the World Health Assembly who endorsed the resolution on "Health for all by the year 2000," confirmed PHC as the central thrust.

- It is applicable in developed as well as in developing countries, and in affluent as well as in poor societies.

4. Requirements for implementation of the plan

   High-authorities support and commitment
   Financial resources
   Administrative reforms
   Health personnel
   Community participation
   Sectoral coordination

Links to a medical school

High-authorities Support and Commitment

The coverage of the Kingdom by a network of primary health care has already been considered as one of the main goals of the health sector in the third five year plan (1401-140-5 AH/1981-1985 AD). What is needed is a common understanding of the objectives and functions of PHC among the high authorities.

In the country at the present time (1984) there are more than 1,500 health centers whose functions are mostly curative.

To turn all or the majority of these health centers into comprehensive healthcare centers is not possible. A more realistic plan is to start with selected PHC units as a model to help in defining the best formula for Saudi Arabia, prior to the propagation of the idea to the rest of the country during the next one or two decades. The proposed PHC in Turaba could serve as one of these pioneering models. The other models could be established in other areas of the country, preferably attached to the medical schools.

The understanding, support and commitment of the health authorities, particularly in the Ministries of Health, Planning and Finance in Riyadh and at the regional level are essential to the success of the plan. This support would facilitate both the provision of adequate financial resources to the PHC as well as administrative reform.

Financial Resources

The budget allocated to the Ministry of Health alone was SR 10,742,000,000. At least 80 percent of this budget presently goes to hospital services, whereas almost 80 percent of the health problems in a developing country like Saudi Arabia could be adequately met at PHC level. What is required is a correction of the disproportionate allocation of the health budget. The additional resources for PHC should be utilized not only by increasing the number, but even more important to improve their quality through:

(a) Improving the quality of the health personnel and preparing them to meet the health needs of the people.

(b) Designing and building a new type of health center which would suit the purpose. Most of the present health centers and dispensaries are accommodated in rented buildings. "The health team in a village in Qasim, when moved to a newly established health center, made an improvement in its activities over the health team in an adjacent village which remained in the old mud housel"

(c) Conducting operational research in health administration. Administration is the bottle neck in the success of health projects.

The community itself should contribute to the PHC both through donations and also by paying fees for services. The additional income should be utilized for continuing improvement of the center.

Administrative Reform

The recent economic prosperity in the Kingdom has led to changes in almost all aspect of life: education; urbanization, _housing and so forth. The health services have expanded greatly in the last decade. A new line of thought should be adopted to handle the changes in the health needs and demands.

In 1978 more than 200 physicians attended two-week courses in community medicine. Apparently the courses did not change their practice since they went back to work within the same system and the same environment. At the end of one of the courses, the 25 participants were asked; "What does a PHC physician need to improve his work?" The majority indicated that he needs a sense of belonging.

PHC in Turaba should be given adequate autonomy in a sense that the leading physician and his team should be involved in the planning as well as the operation of activities. This will give them a feeling of responsibility and self respect and it should be done in accordance with a dual referral system which ensures standardization, supervision and follow-up from the regional director of health services in Taif.

Health Personnel

A major obstacle facing PHC in Saudi Arabia is the quality of the health personnel. The physical resources are almost sufficient if utilized efficiently and so is the number of health personnel, if appropriately used. The quality of most of the health personnel including their training, education, motivation, ability to communicate and leadership capacity needs to be improved.

The majorities of health personnel in Saudi Arabia are, and will remain for many years to come, expatriate. Many of them do not speak Arabic and are not oriented to the health ecology and health problems in the Kingdom.

In the case of Turaba, the three physicians and the dentists are all expatriates which hinders their leadership capacity, even if they have that quality. This stems mostly from the culture which expects the expatriates to follow the rules rather than to innovate. Two of the physicians are non-Arabs, which limits their ability to communicate with other health workers and the community.

One would expect from physicians working in a PHC set-up, to be adequately educated in the area of:

- Ecology of health, which interrelates between health per se and the socioeconomic and environmental factors.

- Primary health care concept, philosophy, objectives and techniques.

- The role of the physician as a leader, educator, clinician and health promoter.

- The role of the community as a primary participant in the health services system.

Unfortunately the classical system of medical education prevailing at the present time in most parts of the world does not sufficiently prepare physicians to play their proper role in PHC. The same would apply to other members of the health team.

The strategy to overcome the problem could be carried out in two phases:

Short Plan:

1. Conducting refresher courses and on-the-job training for all categories of health workers in the objectives, functions and activities of PHC.

2. Better selection in the recruitment of personnel to the system.

Long Term Plan:

1. Establish a higher institute for postgraduate education in family and community medicine in Saudi Arabia to train leaders in the health services system.

2. Support and promote the new trend in medical education being realistically adopted by the present medical schools. The new trend calls for a community-based, problem-solving approach.

Community Participation

This is an issue of utmost importance. The community should participate in all activities of the PHC, defining the problems, planning, implementation, follow-up and evaluation. Also it should contribute to its physical and human resources. School teachers and pupils, religious leaders and many other individuals and groups can be involved.

Section VII of the declaration of Alma Ata states that PHC "requires and promotes maximum community participation in the planning, organization, operation and control of primary health care making fullest use of local, .natural and other variable resources."2 The concept has also been highlighted in the preceding conference held in Halifax, May 1978 on" Primary Health Care: A Global Perspective, the Role of Non-Governmental Organization."

The seven countries participated in a study on "Country Decision Making for the Achievement of the Objective of Primary Health Care" indicated that community participation is vital for the success of PHC.

Turaba itself can give an example of the readiness of the people to participate in public projects. The people of Ergain, under the leadership of their sheikh donated two small houses for the school and the dispensary, paved part of the road to Souq and introduced electricity to their village. Our experience in the field supports this self-reliant attitude among rural communities.

In Tamnia village, the school children and their teachers contributed to the cleanliness of their village.4 In Qasim village school children and their teachers were activated to carry out a program of Trachoma control, health education and vaccination in their community.5 Through ARAMCO medical department, Saudi Arabia, a reduction of diarrheal diseases in children was achieved by the introduction of "day care" programs with the participation of the mothers.

Community participation can also be expressed by paying nominal fees for outpatient service. The government of Saudi Arabia is determined to provide its people with appropriate health care facilities. The principle of applying nominal fees for certain aspects of health services has already been accepted by the authorities in response to the first national development plan. It is expected to give better recognition of the health services from the part of the people, emphasize the contribution of the community and help in cutting off some of the unnecessary load on the health facilities. The income from the fees should be put at the disposal of the health care center to initiate community based projects and carry out general improvements.

Community participation in physical, human and moral forms will build up self-reliance, self-identification with the health projects and a feeling of belonging. The village committee or likewise, if strong and motivated, can give the initiative for community participation.

Sectorial Coordination

Health promotion is beyond the capacity of the health sector alone. Various government sectors such as the departments of agriculture and municipality should cooperate with the health sector: The Development Center with its four sections- health, agriculture, education and social welfare- can work as a base for such coordination.

Links to a Medical School

The PHC will function as a base for training programs in family medicine practice, health administration, and a wide range of preventive programs. On-the-job training, short courses, symposia and conferences can be held for health personnel from the region.

The links of the pioneering PHC centers with medical schools would facilitate, to a great extent, the education and training programs. Research will also be promoted. The idea of connecting PHC to educational institutions has been implemented successfully in Rockford School of Medicine, University of Illinois College of Medicine, University of Washington School of Medicine, Bu Ali Sina University, Hamadan, Iran, University of Glasgow, Hacettepe University, Turkey, and in Kenya.

BIBLIOGRAPHY

1. Sebai ZA. Ed. Community Health in Saudi Arabia: A Profile of Two Villages in the Qasim Region. Saudi Medical Journal Monograh No.1. Great Britain: Stanhope Press, 1982.

2. WHO/UNICEF Primary Health Care Report; Alma Ata, USSR: September 1978.

3. UNICEF/WHO. National Decision Making for Primary Health Care. Geneva, WHO, 1981 (UNICEF/WHO JC 23).

4. Sebai ZA, El Hazmi MA, Serenius F. Health Profile of Preschool Children in Tamnia Villages, Saudi Arabia. Saudi Medical Journal, 1981; 2 (Suppl. 1): 68-71.

5. Sebai ZA. Ed. Community Health in Saudi Arabia: A Profile of Two Villages in the Qasim Region. Saudi Medical •Journal Monograph No. 1. Great Britain: Stanhope Press, 1982.

6. ARAMCO Epidemiology Bulletin. Aramco Medical Department, Dhahran, Saudi Arabia. June/ July 1974.

7. Pittman J, Daniel MB. Undergraduate Education in Primary Care; The Rockford Experience. Journal of Medical Education, 1977; 52: 982-90.

8. Gordon MJ, et al. Evaluation of Clinical Training in the Community. Journal of Medical Education, 1977; 52: 888-95.

9. Villareal R. Health Services and Manpower Development Program, Iran, Hamadan and West Azerbaigan Provinces. Geneva, WHO, 1977 (WHO Assignment Report. EM/HMD/383).

10. Hannay DR, Maddox EJ. The Use and Perception of a Health Center. Practitioner, 1977; 218: 260-66.

11. Fisik N. Professor of Community Medicine, Hacettepe University, Ankara, Turkey (personnal communication).

12. Fendall NE. Paper Presented at Rural Health Conference of the South Pacific Commission, Tahiti, April 1963.

13. Fendall NE. et al. A National Reference Health Center for Kenya. East African Medical Journal, 1963; 40 (4).

The Role of Hospitals In Training Health Professionals for Primary Health Care

This article has three objectives: first to discuss some features of the role of hospitals in training and orienting health personnel to primary health care (PHC); second to review why this role is not adequately fulfilled and third to draw up some guidelines for improvement.

The subject is too broad and diverse to be wholly covered in this section. The material presented here is based on personal experiences in Saudi Arabia and some of the countries in the Mediterranean region and is meant to serve as a baseline for discussion and a stimulant for other ideas and thoughts. Let us begin by stating the problem: hospitals have a great potential within their human physical resources to promote the training of health personnel in PHC. Unfortunately they are not fulfilling this role. The reasons are many and they can always be traced back to the failure of traditional medical education to train and orient health authorities and professionals in the concept of primary health care.

The features of the traditional medical education system are predominantly hospital based, curative medicine oriented, teacher centered and physician patient relationship oriented.

This is quite different from what is needed in the training of physicians and other health workers to deliver comprehensive care to improve the health of the individual, the family, and the community. In most countries the pattern of health services delivery systems is predominantly curative and the relationship between primary, secondary and tertiary levels of care is distorted. The budget allocation and the administrative support given to the three levels of care are unbalanced and a dichotomy between health services and health manpower development prevails.

Primary Health Care

What is PHC? The Alma Ata conferences described the health care aspects of PHC as "essential health care, based on practical, scientifically sound and socially acceptable methods and technology, made universally acceptable to individuals and families in the community through their full participation and at a cost that the community and the country can afford to maintain at every stage of their development, in the spirit of self-reliance and self determination." The eight tasks enumerated in the declaration of Alma Ata as the minimum core of PHC are:

1. Health education
2. Food supply and nutrition
3. Water and basic sanitation
4. Maternal and child health and family planning
5. Immunization
6. Communicable disease control and prevention
7. Basic curative care
8. Essential drugs

PHC became the main theme in health care in the last few years and almost every health authority can easily articulate the wording of its objectives and functions. Nevertheless, the practice of PHC (all over the world) is still mainly to provide curative and palliative medicine to the attending outpatients. The main reason for this is the type of medical education received by the authorities and the health personnel working in PHC.

The Role of Hospitals

Hospitals constitute resource centers for training all categories of health manpower. Whereas 80 percent of the health problems of the community could be adequately met by PHC, the hospitals' share of the health services budget is 80 percent or greater. The secondary care hospitals in particular are by their nature in a position to strengthen the links between PHC and tertiary care, between advanced biomedical research and practice and the "grassroots" of the health problems of the community, and between medical schools and the health services system.

The training of PHC personnel could be supported and enhanced by hospitals in a variety of ways.

1. Undergraduate Education and Training

    Ministry of Health hospitals (local district and regional) as well as
    university hospitals should be properly utilized in training physicians
    and other health professionals. A new and growing concept of medical
    education calls for an early and balanced exposure of students to clinical
    medicine, epidemiology and family and community health. Training
    can take place in the hospital ward and outpatient departments, health
    centers and health posts, in lecture rooms and the community as a
    whole. Whenever possible training should bring together the various
    members of the health team.

2. Postgraduate Education

    Hospitals could play a major role in postgraduate education if they
    were properly oriented.

    The postgraduate programs in family medicine, general practice and
    other clinical specialties in the western world are modeled to suit their
    health needs and there is still room for improvement. The schools
    of public health have generally been criticized for being separated
    from clinical sciences. We hope that the residency programs in the
    developing world, particularly in the area of family health and general
    practice, will be tailored to relevant needs and emphasize the holistic
    approach to health.

3. Continuing Education

    Hospitals can take positive action in promoting continuing education.
    This can be in the form of on-the-job training, refresher courses,
    symposia, conferences, and the preparation of educational materials
    for self and distant learning (television and radio programs, tape
    recordings, transparencies, films and newsletters). The programs
    of continuing education can encompass the eight tasks of PHC
    recommended by the Alma Ata conference along with the practical

aspects of epidemiology and health management including group dynamics and team leadership.

Educational programs are to be directed to health professionals (who are the prime target) as well as to health authorities, educators, directors of other sectors related to health, and community leaders. Such programs organized by hospitals can be held in hospitals, the community, the health centers or in the home.

In summary, hospital personnel can play their greatest role as educators, trainers, health promoters and innovators. They need to be prepared to accept this role.

How to Improve the Hospital Role in Training and Orienting Health Personnel towards PHC.

A prerequisite for the improvement is to promote understanding, willingness and commitment. As has been stated previously, health authorities and educators in many developing countries, influenced by the global awareness, have begun talking about PHC. But their actual understanding, willingness and commitment is currently less than evident.

Firstly, there is a need for reorientation. Secondly a new generation of health personnel with fresh and attitudes is required to apply the message before the year 2000 is on the doorstep - and yet we are still talking about PHC. It must also be recognized that attaining the goal 'Health for all' is the responsibility of all who deal with socioeconomic development and not those in the health sector alone.

The improvement of the role of hospitals towards. PHC can possibly be achieved in two ways: reorientation of health authorities and hospital personnel and improving medical education.

A.   Reorientation of Health Authorities and Hospital Personnel

This needs to be a well conceived and directed plan to reorient all personnel involved in hospital practice, i.e. decision makers, planners, educators, regional health directors, directors of hospitals and physicians working in hospitals. It would also include authorities of other related sectors and community leaders. The reorientation program should be directed to improve knowledge, attitudes and practice of authorities and hospital physicians. towards the concept, function and effectiveness of PHC. The program can be implemented in a variety of ways including group discussion, conferences, study tours, etc., but the best approach is to demonstrate a mode where a hospital is involved successfully in teaching of PHC personnel.

The ultimate goals of the orientation program are:

a.   To gain the understanding and support of health authorities for the importance of PHC. This should lead to:

- Realignment of the disproportionate allocation of health budgets,

- Administrative reform to give adequate autonomy for hospitals and PHC centers and to involve them in planning as well as operation,

- Strengthening the links between primary, secondary and tertiary care, and the links between the health care system and the medical education institutes.

b.   To promote understanding, willingness and commitment of hospital personnel to participate in and promote the training of PHC personnel. The process of reorientation of health authorities and hospital personnel takes time and effort, but it is the starting point before any real achievement can be hoped for in involving hospitals in training and orienting PHC personnel.

B.   Improving Medical Education

This is the most effective and lasting way to improve the role of the hospitals in promoting PHC. Medical education should be relevant to the needs and demands of the people. This requires innovative changes in the institutional and educational objectives, curriculum content and methods of learning in the present traditional medical schools.

New approaches have to be established. There should also be full utilization of available resources, mainly the community resources and the Ministry of Health and hospitals and other facilities. In some countries medical schools have become responsible for health services delivery. This would strengthen the relationship between medical schools, the community, and the health services system, help in orienting medical education to the actual health needs, and stimulate basic and applied research. It would also lead to a better awareness of hospitals of their function as health promoters rather than as mere curative institutes.

There are many innovative features of curriculum design widely accepted in the world as medical education. Each medical school curriculum should reflect its country's particular situation. These features as they differ from the traditional system include:

- Community orientation,

- Problem solving approach,

- Integrated, multidisciplinary teaching,

- Student centered approach,

- Self learning,

- Balanced exposure to clinical medicine, health ecology, epidemiology and behavioral sciences.

The graduates of the community-oriented medical schools, schools of public health and training institutions for health assistants will, in their future capacities as leaders, planners, educators and practitioners, enhance the positive and active role of hospitals in training and orienting of physicians and other health professionals towards primary health care.

Medical Education in Saudi Arabia Which Way Forward?

During the past two decades the important role of medical education has gained recognition not only among the medical profession but also among other health professionals. Whether schools be "traditional" or "innovative" most are involved in the continuing process of curriculum evaluation.* Is the curriculum fulfilling the aims and goals of the school? Does it provide the efficient learning experience for the student? Are the teaching methods effective? Do the assessment procedures provide appropriate information?

The concepts of medical education that are recognized and described around the world should also be considered in Saudi Arabia. Saudi medical education should examine these concepts carefully to determine how they should be applied and the direction of future development. Should there be a single curricular model for the Kingdom or should each school develop independently? Should Saudi schools maintain a "traditional" approach or should they follow the lead of more "innovative" schools? Is there a unique national pattern which can be developed to meet our own needs? Can we adapt and modify some of these advances in medical education? In general there is an urgent need for a new approach to medical education for there is a widespread, if not clearly articulated, dissatisfaction with the traditional or conventional curricula.

Abrahamson1 identified nine diseases of the curriculum: curriculosclerosis, carcinoma of the curriculum, curricula arthritis, curriculum disesthesia, iatrogenic curriculitis, intercurrent curriculitis, curriculum hypertrophy, idiopathic curriculitis and curriculum ossification.

Not one school suffers from all these problems but in most schools many are prevalent, often to such an extent as to handicap the declared aims and goals of the schools. The western model of medical education has been widely copied and adopted throughout the world and the Middle East is no exception. As a consequence, a gap has developed between the training provided for physicians and the real health needs of the countries. In short, in many places medical education may be prescribed as irrelevant and isolated and as a consequence there is a risk that it could become discredited.

Examples are readily available. Throughout the Middle East infectious diseases, malnutrition, inadequate sanitation and inappropriate socioeconomic and cultural conditions are the major factors causing health problems. Traditional medical schools follow curricula which do not prepare their graduates for these problems.

Studies of health centers in Saudi Arabia2, Yemen3 and Oman4 revealed that the function of the physician in the health center was very limited for he saw himself only in a curative role. He waited for the sick to present themselves to him and saw no role in extending health care beyond the walls of the health center, or in providing comprehensive health care. There was little or no evidence of a team approach to health problems or any community participation. The strongest reason for the attitudes and perception of the health problems displayed by these physicians was the influence of their medical education.

In general, health service provision retains a strong curative bias. Progress is measured by the number of physicians produced or by the beds made available, rather than by improvement in the morbidity or mortality rates. The policy makers responsible for this are the products of the traditional schools.

In a study of the central hospital of the Qasim region of Saudi Arabia, the bed occupancy rate was found to be 50 percent. Unfortunately the principles of management and the appropriate utilization of resources to meet health problems had not been covered in medical schools. Now there is a desire for change, to innovate and meet the real challenges to health that our people face. But we must be careful not to repeat the same mistakes of the past. It would indeed be ironic if once again we set out to copy and did not first stop to think and evaluate. Of course we must learn from experiences elsewhere. There is much we have to consider - some ideas to adopt, some to modify, but we have a tale to tell and ideas-to contribute. The more we are able to develop our own ways the richer will be our contribution. For all of us, medical education is a dynamic and continuing process.

The Chances in Saudi Arabian Medical Education.

The birth of medical education in Saudi Arabia came with the establishment of the first medical college at King Saud University, Riyadh, in 1969. At first this college was affiliated to the University of London and its associated medical schools. This affiliation had a considerable influence on the curriculum- its content and the approaches to learning. In many ways it was a typical traditional western curriculum. It was hospital based, curative oriented and the teaching, which was essentially didactic, was undertaken by departments or disciplines.

Some features of the curriculum illustrates these points. Only 120 hours were given to studying the health problems of the nation and none were taught before the fourth year. Further, the teaching was completely restricted to the college and there was no provision for the community experience. In

1975 the college council was asked to consider a proposal to take 20 students for one week of experience in the community. The initial response was rejection for it was believed that time so spent would be at the expense of the more important hospital training and experience. Later, somewhat reluctant approval was given to give the proposal a trial.

The establishment of two more colleges of medicine in 1975, King Abdulaziz at Jeddah and King Faisal in Dammam, coincided with a growing international awareness and increased interest in the important role of medical education. The influence of this may be traced to some extent in the subsequent development of these colleges. Both have accepted the wider responsibility of producing ultimately other members of the health team. Their aims and objectives and educational philosophy have shown some commitment towards community orientation and integration.

In the past decade many international meetings have focused on the new concepts of medical education and in particular the necessity of increasing the relevance of educational programs to the needs of the people – Tehran (1978), Nova Scotia (1978), Alma Ata (1978), Washington (1981) and Karachi (1982). In 1977, a "network" of medical schools was established with a commitment to promote community-oriented medical education programs and a problem-solving approach to learning. New and innovative medical schools emerged - McMaster in Canada, Newcastle in Australia, Maastricht in the Netherlands, Gezira and Juba in Sudan, Suez Canal in Egypt and many others in both the developing and developed world. They pioneered significant advances in many areas of medical education and their contributions are now widely acknowledged.

In 1980, a fourth medical college was established in Saudi Arabia at Abha in the southwestern region. By this time the vital and changing role of medical education had gained universal recognition. The World Health Organization and other national and international agencies had identified the importance of primary health care as a method for providing better and more relevant health care to the needs of developing and developed nations alike. Medical education had now the responsibility for producing physicians who could contribute or relate to the health problems of the individual, the family and the community.

In planning the medical college at Abha, an attempt was made to examine many of these advances and take them into account in designing the educational program (see pp. 228- 232).

In the three other Saudi medical schools there are also signs of change. At Riyadh, after the initial rejection of the proposal to provide a community experience for students, field trips have been organized on a regular basis since 1975. They became so popular with staff and students that in 1980, 40 staff members wished to join us on the field trip. Other advances include planning for satellite health clinics for both family medicine and primary health care and the training of medical students. A department of medical education has been established.

At Dammam the Department of Community Medicine is fast becoming one of the largest in the college.

In Jeddah, a teacher-training program and a continuing education program for allied health personnel has been started. Integrated assessment techniques are being tried and symposia on integrated teaching have been held.

Joint boards have been established between the Ministry of Health, Medical Services Departments in the Ministry of Defense and the National Guard, and the three medical colleges to promote continuing education programs and postgraduate training.

Postgraduate residency programs in surgery, medicine, pediatrics, obstetrics and gynecology and family medicine have commenced in the colleges of medicine under the umbrella of the Arab Boards for Medical Specializations. In the first Saudi Medical Conference in 1976, minimal time was given to preventive medicine and practically no time to medical education. During the past several years there has been a radical change and now whole sections of annual conferences are devoted to preventive medicine and medical education.

The Riyadh, Jeddah, Dammam and Abha are medical schools utilizing the facilities of the Ministry of Health and the Armed Forces for teaching. Agreements between the Colleges of Medicine and the Ministry of Health permit the colleges to have access to all health service units in their regions for teaching purposes. These are all indications of the progressive interaction between medical education programs and health care systems.

Conclusion

The first three medical colleges in the country started with conventional and traditional educational programs. They are now developing more innovative approaches. The College of Medicine at Abha is in harmony with the other three and aims to relate its curriculum to the health needs of the country.

Advances and developments in medical education are essential and must occur. There can be no better investment for Saudi Arabia than to provide high quality physicians and other health personnel who are trained to meet the health needs of the country today and tomorrow.

More changes and more ideas will continue to develop within the four colleges. Inevitably, each will develop its own identity. They will not resemble each other, and neither should they. Each must keep abreast of new developments in medical education and learn from national and international experience.

7

REFERENCES

1. Abrahamson S. Diseases of the Curriculum. Journal of Medical Education 1978; 53: 951-957

2. Sebai ZA., Miller D. and Ba'Ageel H. A Study of Three Health Centres in Rural Saudi Arabia. Saudi Medical Journal 1980; 4: 197-202.

3. Sebai ZA. Health Manpower Development in Yemen Arab Republic 1976; WHO Assignment Report No. EM/HMD/359.

4. Sebai ZA. Health Manpower Development in Oman 1978; WHO Assignment Report No. EM/HMD/394.

5. Moustafa AT. Hospital Services in the Qasim Region with Emphasis on Breida General Hospital. In: Sebai Z, ed. Community Health in Saudi Arabia, Saudi Medical Journal Monograph No. 1, MacMillan Publishers Ltd., 1982: 77-86.

A New Faculty of Medicine at Abha

"Life is short, and art long, occasion instant, experiment perilous decision difficult." - Hippocrates

In 1980, a new faculty of medicine was established at Abha, the capital of the southwestern region of Saudi Arabia (Figure 7 p. 29). The decision was based on a study conducted in 1977 which indicated that to increase the number of Saudi physicians from 318 (8 percent of the total in Saudi Arabia in 1977) to

3,567 (50 percent of the total projected for 1980), it was necessary to open a new medical school, the fourth in the country.

The health services system in the developing world, including those of the eastern Mediterranean region, reflect the following pattern: an emphasis on curative services and the physician-patient relationship, meeting demands rather than actual needs; a lack of a health team approach; inadequate community participation and insufficient integration between health and socioeconomic development. These features have largely resulted in a failure to tackle the roots of the•health problems at individual, family or community levels.

Several studies of the health care system in Saudi Arabia have shown some indications of irrelevancy to health needs and under-utilization of health resources. These features are common in developing countries and are not peculiar to Saudi Arabia.

The main determining factor causing this inept pattern of health services is the type of medical training and orientation given to physicians during their medical studies. Traditional medical education, mostly copied from the western world is hospital-based, curative medicine oriented and teacher centered. This has affected to a great extent the attitudes, behavior and practice of physicians in their roles as health planners, policy makers, educators, administrators and medical practitioners.

Many newly established medical schools, tried to find an answer to the question of relevancy and competency, by introducing a variety of approaches in their programs. Harrell and Vann (1945) called for interdepartmental correlation, a breakdown of artificial preclinical/clinical barriers and the planning of the scattered phases of medicine as one coherent whole. Other ideas have followed including a problem-solving approach in learning and practicing medicine; the integration of medical preparation with the preclinical medical sciences; the scientific rationale of medicine; relating the curriculum to student needs and interests with an integrated basic sciences program; the development of the medical school as a sociocultural institution; and the direction of medical education towards national health needs, entailing the integration of clinical disciplines into community health programs.

It is imperative that we in Saudi Arabia do not delay efforts to improve ways and means to educate and train physicians and other health workers to be better prepared to meet our health needs.

The Community

The Southwest Region has a high population density. The 1,001,640 people represent approximately 20 percent of the total population of the Kingdom. About 75 percent live in rural areas and are engaged in agriculture, trade and government employment. Fishing and animal husbandry are pursued to a lesser extent.

The area is one of the most scenic and breathtaking in the Kingdom. It stretches from the town of Al Nimas, south of Taif, to the frontier with North Yemen. To the west bordering the Red Sea there is a narrow coastal plain (Tihama). Running down the center there is a chain of rugged mountains extending up to 9,000 feet high, in which live a variety of tribes described by the explorer Wilfred Thesiger as "a graceful laughing people." To the east the land slopes away to plains and open desert.

Health services are less than average for the nation. Out of 640 Saudi physicians (1980), only three are working in the region. The infant mortality rate is over 100 per 1,000 live births. 13In general there is a higher prevalence of health problems in the southwest than in the rest of the country, especially in the lowlands of Jizan, Najran and Tihama. These include gastroenteritis, malnutrition and pneumonia among children, as well as malaria, schistosomiasis, tuberculosis, endemic syphilis (bejel), and leishmaniasis. Cases of leprosy, filariasis, onchoceriasis and visceral leishmaniasis have also been reported.

Objectives of the Faculty

In the initial planning stage, the objectives of the faculty were laid down.

Institutional Objectives

1. Education: to produce physicians and ultimately other members of the health team capable of promoting health in Saudi Arabia.

2. Research: to promote basic and applied scientific research in the Southwest Region.

3. Services: to participate with the Ministry of Health, the community and other related agencies in the improvement of health services in the region.

Educational Objectives

1. To train high caliber physicians who are: (a) knowledgeable and skilled in providing comprehensive health care (curative, preventive and promotive) and will consider the family as the unit of society; (b) capable of pursuing their postgraduate education in any specialty to an international standard; (c) members of the health team, with leadership capacity; (d) health promoters with a positive role in improving and maintaining the health of the people; and (e) self-learners with responsibilities for continuing their own education. •

2. To train other members of the health team.

3. To create educational models through programs of continuing education for all health personnel.

4. To activate community participation in planning and implementation of health services programs.

Strategy of Development

The preparatory phase of development lasted from October 1980 until May 1981 and was devoted to carrying out preliminary studies, consultations and general planning. Twenty-one medical schools in Saudi Arabia, the United States, Canada, Britain, The Netherlands, Sri Lanka and Kuwait were visited to explore their objectives, educational approaches, innovations and orientation of their medical programs and to seek opportunities for cooperation.

At the same time a series of short consultation meetings of five to seven days duration were held at Abha, to which participants were invited from different countries together with their counterparts from the three Saudi faculties of medicine and the Ministry of Health. The groups represented a variety of disciplines (deans of new and old schools of medicine, educators, planners and practising physicians) and diverse cultural and methodological philosophies, but all had a common interest in medical education. Consultants with backgrounds in architecture, health administration and budget analysis were also present. These meetings helped us to verify our objectives, to define the plan of action, to discuss the physical plan, to study organizational structure and staffing requirements and gradually to develop the curriculum outline.

Curriculum Design

In the development stage, the curriculum becomes a major task for it must reflect the objectives and philosophy of the faculty and determine its overall planning. As we are ready to accept the challenge of producing medical graduates of a high caliber who are adequately oriented to meet the health problems of Saudi Arabia, this requires that the curriculum be related to the existing as well as the future needs of a country which is experiencing a rapid and progressive change in socioeconomic and cultural aspects of its life as well as in the health needs and demands of its people. Also, the need for systematic planning, flexibility, appropriate selection of key personnel and consistent revision and feedback must be recognized.

Features of the curriculum include:

1. Secondary-school graduates with 12 years basic education, both male and female, will be accepted into the six-year program leading to MB BS and followed by one year of internship. Selection of the students will depend on their secondary school grades and their abilities, interests and personal merits.

2. In the first two years, the English language and natural and behavioral sciences will be studied. Early contact with the Saudi environment and human ecology will be emphasized.

3. Exposure to the practice of health, with family attachments in urban and rural societies, posts in primary health care units, community projects and hospital work assignments will take place from the first year.

4. Self-learning skills will be developed through the use of learning resource materials (library, current literature and audiovisual aids), group discussions and electives.

5. Family medicine will bridge the artificial gap between curative and preventive medicine to promote and maintain optimum health. Preventive aspects of medicine wilr tie taught within the sphere of every subject including microbiology, pathology, behavioral sciences, family and general medicine, pediatrics, gynecology and obstetrics, ophthalmology, etc. This will be in addition to courses in health ecology, epidemiology, sanitation, health administration and research methodology including problem-solving.

6. Correlation and integration, both vertical and horizontal, through interdisciplinary courses, synchronization of timing, group discussions and seminars, joint appointments of staff, etc. are significant components in the curriculum design.

Contemporary Activities

Along with curriculum development, other activities have taken place including: establishing a base for the faculty at Abha and formulating a small nucleus of permanent administration and key faculty members; continuing the contacts with the educational institutions inside and outside the Kingdom; signing agreements with the Ministry of Health and Ministry of Defense and Aviation for mutual cooperation with their health resources in the Southwest Region; conducting relevant studies, e.g. the health manpower situation in the Southwest Region, organizing a library and other educational resources.

By early May, 1981, an operational budget had been approved for the faculty to recruit personnel and conduct basic research. A capital budget to design and construct the natural sciences building, which is to serve as the first phase of the ultimate physical facilities, was also approved. Preliminary architectural planning for development of the site and buildings for the next phase of construction continues.

The faculty became a parallel second college of medicine as part of King Saud University in May 1981, at the end of the preliminary planning phase. Further development of the curriculum, verification of the objectives, and augmentation of ways and means to implement our goals in education, research and health services continue.

REFERENCES

1. Khogali A, Mejia VA and ldris AI. Manpower Development in Saudi Arabia. WHO Report 1978; EM/HMD/389.

2. Miller DL and Sebai ZA. In: Proceedings of the 5th Saudi Medical Meeting, Riyadh, 1980. Ed. E.S. Mahgoub et al. College of Medicine, Universityof Riyadh; Riyadh; 69.

3. Moustafa AT In: Community Health in Saudi Arabia. Ed. Z.A. Sebai. Saudi Medical Journal 1982; Monograph 1 :77.

4. Harrell GT and Vann HM. Journal of the Association of Medical Colleges 1945; 20: 139.

5. Tosteson DC. New England Journal of Medicine 1979; 301 :690.

6. Gillhorn A. Commonwealth Fund Report 1980; 62:13.

7. Campbell EJM. Lancet 1976; i:134.

8. Williams G. Western Reserve's Experiment in Medical Education and its Outcome. Oxford University Press 1980; 91.

9. DayS. In: Health Communications. Monograph Publication of the International Foundation for Biosocial Development and Human Health, New York: 1979:195.

10. Bryant JH. In: Medical Education and the Contemporary World. Ed. GE Miller. Us DHEW Publication No. (NIH) 77-1232. 1976; 171.

11. Hartley DRW. Saudi Medical Journal 1980; 1:187.

12. Sebai ZA, Miller DL, Ba'aqeel H. Saudi Medical Journal 1980; 1: 197.

13. Sebai ZA, EI-Hazmi MAF, Serenius F. Saudi Medical Journal 1981; 2, Suppl.1:68.

14. Arfaa F. American Journal of Tropical Medicine and Hygiene 1976; 25: 295.

15. Bayoumi RA, Orner A, Samuel APW, Shah N, Sebai ZA, Sabaa HMA. Tropical and Geographical Medicine 1979; 31: 245.

16. Nadim A, Seyedi-Rashti MA. Cutaneous Leishmaniasis in Saudi Arabia. WHO Report 1977 EM/PD/11, EM/CD/16.

17. Saha N, Bayoumi RA, Sheikh FS El, et al. American Journal of Physical Anthropology 1980; 52: 595.

18. Samer 51. In: Proceedings of the 4th Saudi Medical Conference, King Faisal University, Dammam 1980; 104.

19. Sebai ZA, Morsey TA. Journal of Tropical Medicine and Hygiene 1976; 79:89.

20. El Behairy F, Jan M, Kamel A, Orner A. In: Proceedings of the 6th Annual Saudi Medical Meeting, Jeddah, 1981.

21. EI-Hazmi MAF. In: Proceedings of the 6th Saudi Annual Medical Meeting, Jeddah, 1981.

22. Morsey TA, Sebai ZA. Journal of the Egyptian Society of Parasitology 1,975; 4 & 5: 103.

23. Sebai ZA. Saudi Medical Journal 1980; 1:133.

24. Sebai ZA, Morsey TA, El Zawahri M. Castellania 1974; 2:263.

25. Sebai ZA, Shehata MH. Ain Shams Medical Journal 1974; 25:551.

لماذا لا نعلم الطب باللغة العربية ؟

موضوع تعليم الطب باللغة العربية مثار جدل لاينتهي بين مؤيديه ومعارضيه ومن يقف منه موقف الحياد .. أثير الأمر في الجامعة السورية في أول نشأتها مع بداية هذا القرن.. وكان أن اتخذ الأطباء السوريون منه موقفا ايجابيا ومن ثم بدأ تدريس الطب باللغة العربية في جامعة دمشق منذ ٧٠ عاماً وتلتها فيما بعد كليتا الطب في حلب واللاذقية. وفكرت الجامعات المصرية منذ عشرين عاماً في تعليم الطب باللغة العربية وبخاضت تجربة صغيرة ثم تراجعت عنها.

كنت لا ألتفت الى هذا الموضوع بجدية تذكر الى بضع سنوات خلت بل كنت أميل الى معارضته الى أن التقيت باستاذنا الطبيب الأديب الدكتور أحمد محمد سليمان الذي كان استاذا للطب الشرعي بكلية الطب بجامعة الملك سعود بالرياض. كان رعاه الله من دعاة تعليم الطب والعلوم الطبية باللغة العربية فأثار هذا الموضوع بيننا والقى فيه أكثر من محاضرة واتضح لي يومها أن سلبيتي كانت من باب (من جهل الشيء عاداه) وما أكثر ما نعادي من أمور لأننا نجهل وجهات النظر الأخرى فيها.

ومن خلال تدريسي لطلبة السنوات النهائية بكلية الطب بجامعة الملك سعود وجدتهم يحجمون عن النقاش والجدل في مايتلقون من علوم ويميلون الى قراءة الملخصات والمذكرات بدل الكتب والمراجع والبحوث. ووجدت قراءتهم باللغة الانجليزية بطيئة لا تساعدهم على البحث والتنقيب وحديثهم لايخلو من الأخطاء. وعدت بذاكرتي الى الوراء وأنا في المراحل الأخيرة من دراستي الطبية فوجدتني لم أكن أفضل منهم حالاً.. كنت لا أملك أن أناقش ولا أملك أن اقرأ بتوسع ولا حتى استطيع أن أعبر عن نفسي كتابة بلغة انجليزية سليمة ولم أكن وحدي وإنما هي ظاهرة كان يشترك فيها جميع زملائي في الدراسة إلا القليل منهم ممن تعلم في مدارس أجنبية. وبعد أن تخرجنا من كلية الطب وجدت أن البعض منا ممن أكمل دراسته العليا بعد ذلك في جامعات الغرب تحسنت لغته الانجليزية أما الباقون من الأطباء وهم الأكثرية الساحقة فلم تتحسن لغتهم إلا بمقدار ضئيل وظني بهم الى اليوم يعانون من صعوبة البحث والقراءة والكتابة وهى عناصر أساسية في تطوير الطبيب.

اثار هذه الخواطر في نفسي مؤتمر أسبوع العلم الذي حضرته مؤخرا في سوريا واستمعت فيه الى محاضرات في الطب القيت باللغة العربية وناقشت بضعة من المحاضرين والاساتذة والطلبة. وزرت كليتي الطب بجامعة دمشق وجامعة تشرين واستمعت وناقشت أكثر. وازددت اقتناعا عن أي وقت مضى بامكانية تعليم الطب باللغة العربية بل وبضرورة تعليم الطب باللغة العربية.

استمعت الى بضعة من المحاضرات في غاية التخصص ووجدت اللغة العربية قادرة على استيعاب مواضيعها والتعبير عنها. ووجدتهم قد ترجموا الآلاف من المصطلحات الطبية عن اللغات الأوروبية. وفي لقاءات جانبية استمعت الى طلبة يناقشون اساتذتهم فكانوا يعبرون عما في خواطرهم بلغتهم الأم فلا يستعصي عليهم النقاش ووجدت في أيديهم مراجع باللغة العربية لا يعجزون عن قراءتها والالمام بها بسهولة ويسر.

هذه تجربة شخصية لا أريد أن أفرضها على القارىء ولكني أحببت أن أجعلها منطلقا لنقاش فكرة..

لماذا لا نبدأ في تعليم الطب باللغة العربية في عالمنا العربي وعدد سكانه يزيد عن المائة وخمسين مليونا ولدينا حوالي خمسين كلية طب أكثرها يدرس الطب بالانجليزية والبعض يدرسها بالفرنسية أو الايطالية. وأمامنا بلدان صغرى من حيث عدد سكانها مثل السويد والنرويج ودول شرق أوربا واليونان وعشرات غير هذه وتلك من الدول الصغيرة جميعها تدرس الطب بلغتها الأم وفي نفس الوقت يتزود الطالب فيها بلغة أجنبية مثل الانجليزية أو الفرنسية لكي تساعده على متابعة البحوث الطبية. ولنا عبرة فيما فعله اجدادنا حين ترجموا علوم الهند وفارس واليونان الى اللغة العربية ثم مافعله الأوروبيون حين ترجموا كتب العرب الى لغاتهم.

فهل آن لنا أن ندرس علوم الطب بلغة العرب ؟

في الاجتماع الأخير الذي حضره عمداء كليات الطب في دول العالم العربي في الأردن في عام ١٤٠٣هـ أقر المجتمعون ضرورة تعليم الطب باللغة العربية وأوصوا بأن يكون الموضوع الرئيسي في اجتماعهم القادم هو وسائل تحقيق هذا الهدف. الأمر اذن تعدى مرحلة التساؤل هل نعلم الطب باللغة العربية أم لا ؟. وأصبح السؤال هو متى وكيف نبدأ؟

في رأيي أن أحد الوسائل هو تشجيع بل فرض الترجمة والتعريب على مستوى واسع من خلال الجامعات وتوفير جميع الحوافز المالية والأدبية والعلمية لذلك وأن يسن قانون بأن لايرتقي مدرس الطب الى مرحلة الاستاذية قبل أن ينشر مقالات طبية باللغة العربية سواء من تأليفه أو ترجمته بالاضافة الى انشاء مجلات طبية باللغة العربية. وطريق طوله الف ميل يبدأ بخطوة واحدة.

لماذا نتبع مناهج التدريس في كليات الطب الغربية ؟

يقاس الوضع الصحي في أي مجتمع بمقاييس متعارف عليها .. من أهمها معدلات الوفيات والأمراض. فاذا أخذنا على سبيل المثال وفيات الأطفال في دولة ما في العالم العربي نجدها تبلغ مائة في الألف في السنة تقريبا أي أنه من بين كل ألف طفل يولد يتوفى ١٠٠ منهم قبل اكتمال العام الأول من حياتهم في حين أنه في دولة أوروبية مثل السويد تبلغ وفيات الأطفال الرضع ٨ في الالف في السنة. ولو أخذنا مرض السل كمثال آخر لوجدنا أن نسبة المصابين به في بعض المجتمعات العربية تبلغ عشرين ضعف نسبة المصابين به في أمريكا الشمالية.

لاشك أن هناك عوامل كثيرة تؤدي الى وجود هذه الفوارق بين المجتمع العربي والمجتمع الأوروبي أو الأمريكي، منها الوضع الاقتصادي والاجتماعي وظروف البيئة بالاضافة الى الرعاية الصحية المتوافرة.

ونحن هنا لسنا في سبيل عقد مقارنة للرعاية الصحية في المجتمعين الأوربي والعربي، ولكننا نريد أن نقول أن الرعاية الصحية في المجتمع العربي مع كل مايبذل فيها من جهد ووقت ومال لا تتلاءم كثيراً مع طبيعة المشاكل الصحية فيه.

واذا ماسألنا أنفسنا لماذا لا تتلاءم الرعاية الصحية مع طبيعة الاحتياجات والمشاكل الصحية في مجتمعنا العربي نجد أن الجواب يكمن في مناهج كليات الطب لدينا. فبالرغم من الاهتمام الجيد بتدريب الأطباء ومع وجود عشرات الكليات والمعاهد الطبية في بلادنا العربية إلا أن الأطباء في أمتنا العربية يدرسون في كلياتهم مناهج دراسية مستعارة في أغلبها من المدارس الطبية في الغرب. هذه المناهج تركز على العلاج دون الوقاية وعلى التصدي للمرحلة النهائية للمرض بدلاً من الاهتمام ببوادره والحد منه ومن مضاعفاته ولاتهيىء الطبيب للعمل الجماعي ضمن فريق طبي كما أنها لا تهيئه للنظرة الشاملة الوقائية والعلاجية والتطويرية.

كليات الطب في الغرب تركز على تدريب الطالب على علاج المريض ولاتهتم كثيراً بأسباب الوقاية ربما لأن مفاهيم الشعوب وصحة البيئة متطورة لديهم. أضف الى ذلك اختلاف المستويات الاقتصادية والتعليمية. أما في بلادنا فأسباب المرض لازالت تكمن في البيئة وعلينا أن نتناولها من جذورها بأسباب الوقاية والعلاج كما أن علينا أن ندرب طالب الطب على الأخذ على هذه الأسباب مجتمعة.

وكنتيجة حتمية للتعليم الطبي الذي يتم أساساً داخل المستشفيات نجد أن الغالبية العظمى من الأطباء في المجتمع العربي أميل الى العمل في المدينة دون القرية وفي المستشفى دون المركز الصحي ولا نجد إلا قلة منهم يتسع مفهومهم للعمل الجماعي الذي يهدف الى رفع المستوى الصحي للمجتمع وليس فقط الاهتمام بالفرد.

وأول سؤال يتبادر الى الذهن اذا اثيرت فكرة انشاء كلية طب جديدة في العالم العربي أي منهج من

مناهج المدارس الغربية سوف تتبع؟

ولا أحد منا يتساءل .. ولماذا بالضرورة تتبع مناهج كليات الطب عندنا مناهج كليات الطب في الغرب؟ هل أمراضنا هى أمراضهم أو حتى تقاربها؟ هل شعوبنا بادراكها الثقافي والتعليمي مثل شعوبهم؟ هل توزيع سكاننا بين الحضر والريف مثل توزيع سكانهم؟ هل توزيع أعمارنا مثل توزيع الأعمار لديهم؟ هل الامكانيات البشرية والمادية التي لدينا مثل التي لديهم؟ الجواب البديهي على كل هذه التساؤلات هو .. لا.

نحن اذن في حاجة الى الطبيب الذي يتسع احساسه بالمسئولية ليشمل المجتمع ولا يقتصر على الفرد. الطبيب الذي يقبل على العمل في الريف كما يقبل عليه في المدينة. الطبيب الذي تدرب على ادارة الفريق الطبي وتوجيهه والاشراف عليه. الطبيب الذي يسائل نفسه ترى الى أي مدى استطعت ـ مع فريقي الطبي ـ أن أقلل من نسبة الوفيات والأمراض.. وليس فقط كم مريضا عالجت اليوم.

ولكي نحصل على مثل هذا الطبيب، علينا أن نعيد النظر بشكل جاد في مناهج كلياتنا الطبية في العالم العربي.

PROBLEM BASED LEARNING

There are many methods of problem-based learning. Several references are available on the subject including:

Kenneth E. Eble, The Aims of College Teaching, San Francisco, J.ssey – Bass

Publishers, 1983.

Katz FM, Fulop T. Personnel for Health Care: Case Studies of Educational Programmes: World Health Organization- Geneva 1978, Public Health Paper No. 70.

Davies IK. Objectives in Curriculum Design; London: Mcgraw Hill 1976.

Seemingly there is no end of new inventions in the field. The following set of exercises represents one of the methods of problem-based learning. It should stimulate interactions, critical thinking, self-expression, and team work. To obtain the maximum benefit, learners must support their discussions by extensive readings of relevant literature.

It is suggested that after students discuss a selected topic in the book, they respond to the questions at the end of the text in a group session. Preferably this should be guided by an educator who will function as a facilitator rather than a teacher. Some of the answers to the questions can be found in the book while others will need reference to literature.

Learners, in groups, are encouraged to plan for the discussion, select relevant exercises, and divide the tasks among themselves. Each group needs to select, among themselves, on a rotating basis, a coordinator, (never a chairman) who would work as a catalyst to the group, and a rapporteur. A blackboard or an overhead projector would facilitate the discussion. Several field projects are listed. It is suggested that a project be carried out by a team of educators and learners. The objective is to provide an experience in planning, implementation, and documentation of health programs. The scope of a project depends on the available resources and time. Extensive reading, planning, and team spirit are always required.

I. GROUP EXERCISES

Health in the Developing World

Statistics from developing countries state that:

- IMR is high (over 150 per 1 000 in the least developed countries}. A newborn child in certain parts of Africa has only a 50/50 chance of surviving through adolescence.

In your opinion, what are the reasons behind this high mortality rate in developing countries?

- Define infant mortality rate (IMR} and age specific death rate.

- Why is IMR a sensitive index of health?

- Discuss other indices of health.

- What are the main measures to lower IMR in a developing community?

- Discuss the immunization program for early childhood with emphasis on the type of vaccines, schedule of immunization, cold chain and community participation.

- Discuss geography as a determining factor in health.

- Afghanistan, Mali, Egypt, and Barbados, all are developing countries. How do you explain such differences in IMR (Table 2, page 4)7

- Discuss the effect of illiteracy and poverty on morbidity and mortality rates.

- Diarrhea, pneumonia, and malnutrition are the main causes of deaths of children below five years of age. Discuss the synergistic action of the three diseases.

- "If all the knowledge of medicine and public health already available by the 1950s had been effectively applied, most causes of morbidity could have been controlled or even eradicated." Do you agree, disagree, or do you have a different opinion? Accordingly, how do you see the priorities in health research?

- Give examples of the effect of ethnicity on the health status of people.

- Which factor is more important as a determinant of health, heredity or environment? Support your argument with statistics.

- How do you explain the steady decline of tuberculosis in England and Wales, well before the discovery of the causative organism or specific treatment? Support your explanation with historical events.

- How do you calculate life expectancy at birth in a community?

- "Children in less developed countries are short, not because of genetics, but because of poor nutrition." Do you accept this statement? Support your opinion with statistics.

- What does the expression "ecosystem" mean to •you?

- "The effect of economy on health depends on how much it could possibly change the lifestyle of the people." Defend the statement. Give examples from your readings and experience.

- From your experience and readings, refer to cases of lack of utilization of health resources (man, money and management).

- Define the following rates:

Crude death rate   Infant mortality rate
Perinatal mortality rate   Maternal mortality rate

- Discuss Thomas Malthus' theory on population growth.

- Current accelerated population growth will have a negative impact on developing countries or perhaps a positive impact. Would you share in the debate.

- We talk a lot about "the Holistic approach" in health services. Is it an achievable goal? What are the obstacles? How could it be achieved?

- Based on your own experience, discuss the impact of the prevailing systems of medical education on the health services delivery system. What innovations do you suggest?

- "Health auxiliaries can contribute significantly in improving the health of the people". Do you believe in that? Support your points of view by examples from literature.

- From your own experience and readings give examples of successful community-based health programs.

- How could the gap between health needs and demands be narrowed in a community like Turaba?

Turaba

Methodology

- Summarize the general layout of Turaba survey.

- Discuss the differences between:

    a.   Retrospective and prospective studies

    b.   Cross-sectional and longitudinal studies

    Give examples
- What are the differences between sensitive and specific tests? Give examples.

- Discuss the basis of sampling technique (determining the sample size, single random sampling, stratified random sampling).

- Write brief notes on:

    linear regression

    correlation
    standard deviation

    standard error

- Problems of human errors, personal motivations, and lack of reliability and validity of assessment - how can they affect the results of a survey? Give examples.

Family Structure

- Consanguinity is the pattern in many traditional societies. How could this possibly affect the health of the offsprings?

- Discuss the possible effects of early marriage and high parity on the mother and child's health.

- What other causes of abortion can you think of, other than those mentioned by a Bedouin woman?

- How does the size of the family relate to the social, mental and physical well-being of its members?

- Family planning has always been a controversial issue. Did you develop a position for or against it? Support your opinion with statistics.

Nutrition

- Does the data in Table 2, page 47, give you an indication of the possible nutritional problems in a Bedouin community?

- Define the following rates:

  Crude birth rate

  General fertility rate

  Age specific fertility rate

  Gross reproductive rate

- Discuss the possible adverse effects of artificial feeding on the health of a child in Turaba.

- What do you think of goat's milk and camel's milk as possible sources of child nutrition?

- Do you know of any sex-discrimination practices which might affect health in its broad sense?

- What alternatives would you suggest for the introduction of solid food and child weaning in Turaba?

Health Status of Preschool Children

- What human errors could be involved in the figures shown in Tables 5 and 6, pages 51 and 52?

- Use the chi-squared test to detect differences between the three communities in infant deaths (Table 7, page 53).

- Are the rates in Table 8, page 54, prevalence or incidence rates? Why? Define both rates. Give examples.

- Discuss the pathogenesis of hair depigmentation, leg edema, and liver enlargement in a two-year old malnourished child.

- Discuss the etiology, clinical manifestation, line of treatment, and measures of control of infantile beri beri.

- What are the possible causes of conjunctivitis among Turaba children?

- What are the pitfalls in relating height and weight to age in Turaba community? What other alternatives would you suggest?

- Discuss the range of the clinical spectrum of protein-calorie deficiency.

- What could be the causes of the iron deficiency anemia among children in Turaba? Suggest measures of prevention.

- Discuss the malaria situation in Saudi Arabia in terms of the epidemiology of the disease and measures of control.

- Give a brief history of cholera in Saudi Arabia.

- What is the significance of a high prevalence rate of E. coli among preschool children in Turaba?

Changing Turaba

- Socieconomic changes that occur very fast in a community, sometimes insure risk factors. Discuss the issue in relation to Turaba. Support your discussion with evidence drawn from other communities.

- Draw a plan for a longitudinal study to measure infant mortality rate in Turaba community.

- Design a plan to:

    a.   study the magnitude of tuberculosis problem in Turaba, and
    b.   to control the problem.

The Health Center

- The physician in Turaba Health Center sees a patient in 61 seconds. How would you improve the situation?

- Illustrate Tables 12 and 13, pages 65-66, by diagrams. Draw inferences.

- The diagnostic facilities in the health center are not utilized effectively. Why? What do you suggest for improvement?

- The population of Turaba has a high rate of dental morbidity. How could the dentist have contributed to solve the problem?

- Run a preliminary estimate of a cost/benefit analysis of an expanded immunization program (EIP) in Turaba.

- In some countries, local birth attendants are trained to deliver health care to the mother and child. Discuss the feasibility and value of such a program in Turaba.

Khulais

-   Several authors believe that education, services and research in the health field are inseparable components. Is this correct? How does this apply to medical education institutions?

-   Discuss the problem of schistosomiasis in Saudi Arabia in terms of epidemiology and methods of control.

-   Discuss the life cycle, mode of transmission, clinical picture and methods of control of Entamoeba histolytica and Taenia saginata.

-   Discuss the relation between the endemicity of malaria and the prevalence of sickle cell anemia.

-   Compare the functions of the two health centers in Turaba and Khulais.

-   How could the health center in Khulais have progressed in the period 1977-1984?

Tamnia

-   "The health status of preschool children reflects the health conditions of the community as a whole." Verify the statement. Support your arguments with evidence.

-   What is the relevancy of examining children for angular stomatitis and nasolabial seborrhea?

-   If facilities permit for one more anthropometric measurement (page 89), which one would you choose: arm circumference, head circumference, chest circumference or skinfold thickness? Justify your choice.

-   Discuss the etiology, clinical picture, line of treatment and measures of prevention of rna rasm us.

- What are the differential diagnoses of hepatosplenomegaly in a school-age child living in Tamnia7

- Discuss the etiology of stunting and wasting among children. Refer to case studies from literature.

- Interpret the results shown in Table 22 page 94. Discuss the relationship between anemia and parasitic infection.

- Write short notes on:

  thalassemia

  microcytic hypochromic anemia

  vitamin 8 12 deficiency

  protein electrophoresis

- Discuss the etiology, clinical picture and line of treatment of ascariasis. Plan for a control measure in Tamnia.

Qasim

- "Undergraduate education should prepare medical students to be able to educate themselves continuously, think rationally and solve problems in real life situations." You are an educator. How would you implement these theories?

- "Settlement and urbanization can affect the health of the people in different ways." This statement deserves an explanation.

- "The influx of expatriates to the Arab Gulf countries can be a major health issue." Explain the subject.

- What are the implications of girls' education on the structure of the family and the health of the child in a Saudi community?

- What are the direct and indirect effects of an improved economy on community health?

- Traditional medicine is a hot topic of discussion. Can you make it cool with logic and broadness of mind?

The Family Structure

- "There is a wide range of factors within the family setting which has an adverse effect on the health of the preschool child." Discuss the subject.

- What are the differences between cross-sectional and longitudinal studies? Give examples.

- What are the daily nutritional requirements of a pregnant woman and a lactating mother?

- Some health authorities encourage domiciliary deliveries. Where do you stand in the debate? Support your opinion with data.

Family Nutrition

- Family nutrition is determined by several factors. One of them is the income of the family. Discuss the other factors.

- Why are there differences in feeding habits of infants between rural Turaba in 1967 and rural Qasim in 1980?

- "The weaning process is critical for child health and development." Explain why. What does literature say on the subject?

- Divorce is a shocking experience for all parties. Discuss the emotional stresses on young children.

- Draw a graph of a population structure for Khusaiba from (Table 25, p. 113). Analyze the figure.

Health Status of Preschool Children

Invent a local calendar of events for a group of uneducated mothers in a Nomadic community. In Qasim villages, 61.1 percent of the examined preschool children experienced coughing and 26.7 percent had diarrhea during the last month.

> What are the possible etiologies behind the two problems?
> Could one or both problems lead to stunting or wasting of the affected child?
> Discuss the pathogenesis.

- Write short notes on the types and the effectiveness of the following vaccines: Salk, Sabin, BCG and OPT vaccines. •

- In AI Asiah, wasting was most common among children between 12-23 months of age and the percentage of stunted children increased progressively with age (Table 32, page 119). Give an explanation.

- Compare wasting and stunting in Tamnia and AI Asiah (Figure 12, page 92 and Figure 16, page 121). Interpret the differences.

- Draw a plan of urgent action for children affected by severe degrees of wasting and stunting.

Primary Health Care

- Compare the health centers in Turaba and Qasim. Draw a list of recommendations for improvement.

- How could Saudi health personnel be motivated to work in the primary health care system? Discuss obstacles and motivations.

- Illustrate graphically Table 35 p. 124, and Table 36, page 126. Analyze and interpret the data.

- Discuss the possible hazards of indiscriminate drug prescription (Table 36, page 126).

- List the most common health problems of children in Qasim. Draw an outline of the preventive health activities supposed to be delivered by the health center. Define the degree of impact of each activity on the listed health problems. An analytical approach is expected. Be imaginative.

- Compare your results with the present situation in Al Asiah.

- Interpret the follow-up report of Qasim in 1981.

- Centralization versus decentralization is a controversial issue. Debate the subject on the basis of your own experience and readings.

Endemic Syphilis

- Discuss the epidemiology of endemic syphilis.

- Describe the technique of FTA test. Compare the sensitivity and specificity of FTA and VORL tests (Table 2, page 135).

- Consider the seropositive reaction to FTA test in Turaba population. Is it caused by an innocent or a virulent organism? This is an interesting topic for debate.

Cholera in Jizan

- Discuss the epidemiology, the clinical picture, the pathogenesis and the line of management of cholera.

- Which one of the measures mentioned on page 139 is more effective in cholera control? Support your argument by statistics.

- How is the susceptibility to cholera affected by age, sex, ethnicity, previous infection, and nutritional status?

- Present to your colleagues the classical work done by John Snow in studying and controlling the cholera epidemic in London, 1854.

- How do social habits and cultural barriers deter patients or people at risk from receiving appropriate health care? Give examples from your own experience and readings.

- Discuss the effect of immunization and chemoprophylaxis on prognosis of cholera.

- Illustrate graphically the data in Table 5, page 143. Calculate the percentage of co-positivity, co-negativity, and the overall agreement.

Cutaneous Leishmaniasis

- Discuss the epidemiology, the clinical manifestations and the method of control of cutaneous leishmaniasis.

- Discuss the immunological aspect of the disease.

- Describe the most recent techniques in treating leishmaniasis.

- Illustrate graphically the data in Table 9, page 150. What are the possible reasons for the steady increase of the disease?

Filariasis

- Filariasis is caused by a nematode parasite of man. Write a brief note on some of the other important nematodes affecting man in Saudi Arabia. Bring statistics into the discussion.

- Write brief notes on four of the important medical anthropodes: life cycle, breeding habitat, role as a vector, and measures of control.

- Discuss the causes, pathogenesis and management of elephantiasis.

Leprosy

- Discuss the clinical picture, pathogenesis, and line of treatment of leprosy.

- Prepare a plan of control of leprosy in Saudi Arabia.

- Why are the samples in the study, both of the hospital and the community, not representative of the country? How could the sample be made more representative?

- In the Saudi Medical Journal, many articles were published on health subjects in Saudi Arabia. Some of the studies were labeled as representative of the country, but they are not. Pick out those studies.

- Illustrate Table 12, page 161, and Table 13, page 162, with diagrams. Interpret the results.

- How would you integrate leprosy care in primary health care?

- A follow-up report has been written on Hadda Hospital and Khulais Health Center. Discuss the progress made at both sites. If there are differences, discuss the reasons.

Zohair A. Sebai

Hemoglobinopathies

- Discuss the etiology, clinical picture, treatment and measures of prevention of a) G-6-PD deficiency and b) sickle cell anemia.

- Discuss ethnicity as a factor behind sickle cell disease ..

- Discuss the basis of sickling and G-6-PD screening tests.

- "The origin of HbS in Hejaz and Asir seems to be Africa" (Page 173). Discuss the statement and support your argument with evidence.
- Hypothetically extend Table 19, page 176, to include 16 other tribes. ^$alculate the mean, the mode and the median.

- By using audivisual aids, present in 10 minutes the findings of the study.

Health Manpower

- Outline a rational process of health manpower planning in a developing country.

- The uneven urban-rural distribution of health personnel is a disturbing problem in developing countries. In Saudi Arabia, what could be the causes and what are your suggestions?

- Compare the ratio of various categories of health personnel to the population of some developed and developing countries. Relate these ratios to selected health indicies. Interpret the findings.

- Discuss the differences between rational and pragmatic planning.

- Discuss the basics of population census. What are the most important vital statistics to be collected?

- Compare the strategies of health services in the first and the last development plans in Saudi Arabia. Deduce the changes over time.

- Why should the achievements of a comprehensive health care program in Saudi Arabia depend in the first place on the orientation of the faculties of medicine?

- "Health problems must be tackled by health teams." Why? To what extent does the statement reflect the present situation in Saudi Arabia?

- The establishment of 15 health institutions for males and 65 for females seems to be impractical. Explore other approaches.

- Two proposals are competing for a limited amount of money – the establishment of a fifth medical school in the country, or the promotion of programs for training health assistants. Take a stand in front of the Ministerial Cabinet.

- The number of Saudi physicians will increase from an estimate of 900 in 1984 to an estimate of 3,500 in 1990. What are the implications for the health services system? How should the health services system be planned in response?

Health Manpower Study in Qasim Region

- The study of the main hospital in Qasim indicates underutilization. What do you suggest for improvement?

- Illustrate Table 3, page 192, and Table 4, page 192, with Diagrams. Draw inferences.

- In Qasim, 44 percent of the nurses and 33 percent of the technical assistants are Filipinos. Discuss the implications of cultural barriers.

- "The main bottle-neck of the health service delivery system in developing countries is in management and administration." Discuss the statement using local and global examples.

- "Only 3 percent of the health personnel have been through a continuing education program." What kind of continuing education programs would you suggest for physicians and health assistants. Prepare a proposal to the Ministry of Health. The emphasis should be on both content and methodology.

- As a health authority, you are faced with the problems mentioned in Table v7, p. 195. How would you handle these problems?

A Study of Three Rural Health Centers

- Discuss the factors influencing the degree of population attendance to a primary health care unit.

- What could be the contributing factors behind the high infant mortality rate in the areas under the study? Discuss the dicotomy between actual and perceived health needs.

- In Wadiyen and Tamnia no vaccines were given in the last one and onehalf years and 10 years respectively. What could be the reasons behind this failure?

- Practically no organized preventive health services are being offered by the three health centers. This is an area for critical discussion.

- Over a 15-month period Khulais health center reported 418 infectious disease cases {pp. 201-202). The logic behind the figures is questioned.

- It has been stated that the three health centers are not performing their functions as agencies of health promotion. Discuss the reasons.

- Does the case of the Imam in Wadiyen bring to your mind stories on how effective community leaders could be?

- It has been concluded that some progress had been made by the two health centers in Tamnia and Wadiyen, but there is a need for further action. Discuss the issue.

Planning for Primary Health Care in Turaba

- What are the various activities of MCH program?

- What are the categories of personnel who would provide MCH program?

- Primaryhealth care physicians in Saudi Arabia need a sense of belonging. How could this need be fulfilled?

- Elaborate on the term "health ecology."

- What would be the scope of action of a physician in his role as a health team leader?
- What is your understanding of community-based medical education?

- List some of the areas in which the community can help in promoting its own health programs?

- What qualities and skills does the primary health care physician need to acquire in order to coordinate between the various health and health related sectors in his community?

The Last Five Articles

After going through the previous exercises, it is suggested that the students themselves develop questions on the last five articles.

1. The Role of Hospitals in Training Health Professionals for Primary Health Care

2. Medical Education in Saudi Arabia - Which Way Forward?

3. A New Faculty of Medicine at Turaba

4. Why Don't We Teach Medicine in Arabic (Arabic)?

5. Why Should We Follow Western School Curriculum (Arabic)?

II. FIELD PROJECTS

Project I

Develop, as a group, a survey on "Health Personnel Perception of PrimarHealth Care." Define the objective, the target group, the sample size anc methodology. Collect, tabulate, analyze and present the data.

Project 2

Develop a plan of action to improve knowledge, attitudes and practice of family and child nutrition in Turaba.

Project 3

You have the authority and the resources to develop a progressive health program in Turaba. How would you implement the program using the community developed center as a base for your activities.

Project 4

Plan for a household survey on selected socioeconomic indices in the community. Prepare and test the questionnaire. Select and train interviewers, and activate the community. Collect, tabulate, analyze and present the data.

Project 5

Conduct a basic survey on "Health Problems, Resources and Services" at a regional or district level.

Project 6

Conduct a survey in a village to assess the degree of stunting and wasting among preschool children.

Project 7

You are requested to establish basic laboratory services in a health center in your community. Draw the plan including an estimate of the capital and current budgets. Write a manual of procedures.

Project 8

Carry out a project of EPI in a selected community. Make use of health auxiliaries and the community.

Project 9

Parallel projects to Project 8 are suggested for the improvement of health education, environmental sanitation and nutrition.

Project 10

The objective is to promote concepts of primary health care. Organize a symposium on the subject. Invite speakers and an audience from various disciplines.

Project 11

There is extensive literature on Arabic and Islamic medicine, but not very much has been written on the public health aspect. The subject needs your contribution.

Project 12

Supervise a group of undergraduate students in carrying out a selected community-based program.

Project 13

Organize a training program in health education for a selected group of school teachers and social workers.

Project 14

Organize an on-the-job training program for a selected group of health assistants.

Project 15

Organize a recording system in a selected health center. The objective is to monitor health problems for planning, intervention, follow-up and evaluation.

Project 16

Conduct a functional analysis study in a selected health center.

Project 17

Conduct a survey on drug policy in the Ministry of Health or in a region. The report should identify the problem in terms of cost, storing, distribution, utilization, efficiency and effectiveness. •

Project 18

Study the epidemiology of endemic syphilis in a selected Bedouin community. Implement a control program.

Project 19

Study the epidemiology of leishmaniasis in a selected village. Plan and implement a control program.

Project 20

Develop a project to study major health problems during Haj.

Project 21

Study the inpatient and outpatient records in Hadda Hospital. Conduct a field survey for early detection of cases among contacts.

Project 22

In the leprosy hospital in Hadda and the psychiatry hospital in Taif, inpatients pile up unnecessarily because of rules and regulations. Study the situation in order to convince the authorities to change the system.

Project 23

Survey the problem of sickle cell disease in a defined community. Plan and Implement a control program.

Project 24

a. Carry a health manpower survey in a defined geographic area;

b. Design a rational and practical plan of health manpower development in the area under study; and

c. Jointly, with the concerned parties, implement the plan.

Project 25

Evaluate the curriculum of one of the health institutes. Develop a plan of action for improvement. Follow-up and evaluate the implementation.

Project 26

Study dental health in a defined community. Develop a plan of action for dental health promotion. The plan should emphasize reorientation and training of health personnel.

Project 27

Study a defined community for the actual and perceived health needs.

Project 28

Design and implement an MCH program in a defined community.

Project 29

Establish a feasibility study of community payment for services. 258

SOURCES OF THE BOOK

Several chapters in the book are based on published material. The following is a list of these publications:

1. Bayoumi RA, Orner A, Samuel APW, Saha N, Sebai AZ, Sabaa HMA. Hemoglobin and Erythrocytic Glucose-6-Phosphate Dehydrogenase Varients Among Selected Tribes in Western Saudi Arabia. Tropical and Geographical Medicine, 1979; 31: 245-252.

2. EL-Hazmi MAF, Sebai ZA. Laboratory Tests Profile for Preschool Children at Tamnia. Saudi Medical Journal 1981; 2:4. 198-202

3. Miller D, Sebai ZA. Evaluation of Khulais Health Center. In: Mahgoub E.ed. Proceedings of the 5th Saudi Medical Meeting. Riyadh: University, 1980: 69-80.

4. Sebai ZA. Knowledge, Attitude and Practice of Family Planning: Profile of a Bedouin Community in Saudi Arabia. Journal of Biosocial Science 1974; 6: 453-461.

5. Sebai ZA, Morsey TA, El Zawahri M. A Preliminary Study on Filariasis in the Western Part of Saudi Arabia. Castellania 1974; 2: 263-6.

6. Sebai ZA, Shehata MH. Cholera Epidemic in Jizan District, Saudi Arabia. Ain Shams Medical Journal 1974; 25: 551-3.

7. Sebai ZA, Morsey TA, FJ. Treatment of Cutaneous Leishmaniasis with Sodium Stibogluconate (Pentostam) in Saudi Arabia. Journal of Egyptian Pubic Health Association 1975; L-No. 1 : 59-62.

8. Sebai ZA, Morsey TA. Cutaneous Leishmaniasis in Bisha Town, Saudi Arabia. Journal of Tropical Medicine and Hygiene 1976; 79: 89-91.

9.   Sebai ZA. Why Should We Follow Western Style Medical Education (Arabic) AI Majalla AI Arabia 1977; 3: 129-130.

10. Sebai ZA, Baker TD. Endemic Syphilis in a Bedouin Community in Saudi Arabia. Ain Shams Medical Journal 1979; 30-1, 2: 12-17.

11. Sebai ZA, Miller D, Baaqueel H. A Study of Three Health Centers in Rural Saudi Arabia. Saudi Medical Journal, 1980; 1 :4. 197-202-

12. Sebai ZA, An Epidemiological Study of Leprosy and Leprosy Care in Saudi Arabia. Saudi Medical Journal 1980; 1 :3. 133-140.

13. Sebai ZA, Abu Sabaa HM, Shalabi S, Bayoumi RA, Miller D. Health in Khulais Villages, Saudi Arabia - An Educational Project. Medical Education 1981; 15: 310-314.

14. Sebai ZA, EI-Hazmi MAF, Serenius F. Health Profile of Preschool Children in Tamnia Villages, Saudi Arabia. Saudi Medical Journal1981; 2: (Suppl. 1): 68-71.

15. Sebai ZA. The Role of the Hospitals in Training and Re-orienting Physicians and Other Health Professionals Towards Primary Health Care. In: Proceedings of Agha Khan Foundation and W.H.O. Karachi, Pakistan, 1981; 24-26.

16. Sebai ZA, ed. Community Health in Saudi Arabia: A Profile of Two Villages in Qasim Region. London: Stanhope Press, 1982.

17. Sebai ZA. Health Manpower -The Problem Facing Saudi Arabia. Saudi Medical Journal 1982; 3-4: 217-221.

18. Sebai ZA. Cairncross RG. Medical Education in Saudi Arabia: Which Way Forward? In: Proceedings of the Seventh Saudi Medical Meeting. Dammam: King Faisal University, 1982: 3-6.

19. Sebai ZA. A New Faculty of Medicine at Abha. Saudi Medical Journal 1983; 4-1: 77-82.

20. Sebai ZA. The Health of the Family in a Changing Arabia. 3rd ed. Jeddah: Tihama Publication, 1983.

FIGURES

11. Khulais Area in West Saudi Arabia 74

12. Grades of Wasting and Stunting Among Tamnia Children (0-72 months)

13. Hemoglobin Concentration (g/dl) m 257 Preschool Children (Tamnia)

14. Map of AI-Asiah District - Qasim Region

15. Detailed Map of Khusaiba Prepared by School Teachers, A Sign of Community Participation

16. Grades of Wasting and Stunting Among Oasim Children (0-72 months)

17. The Area of the Filariasis Study

18. Areas of Residence of 72 Saudi Leprous Patients